Springer Series on Geriatric Nursing

Mathy D. Mezey, RN, EdD, FAAN, Series Editor

New York University Division of Nursing

1992 **Critical Care Nursing of the Elderly**

   Terry T. Fulmer, RN, PhD, FAAN, and Mary K. Walker, PhD, RN, FAAN

1993 **Health Assessment of the Older Individual, Second Edition**

   Mathy Doval Mezey, RN, EdD, FAAN, Shirlee Ann Stokes, RN, EdD, FAAN, and Louise Hartnett Rauckhorst, RNC, ANP, EdD

1994 **Nurse–Physician Collaboration: Care of Adults and the Elderly**

   Eugenia L. Siegler, MD, and Fay W. Whitney, PhD, RN, FAAN

1995 **Strengthening Geriatric Nursing Education**

   Terry T. Fulmer, RN, PhD, FAAN, and Marianne Matzo, PhD(c), RN, Cs

1996 **Gerontology Review Guide for Nurses**

   Elizabeth Chapman Shaid, RN, MSN, CRNP, and Kay Huber, DEd, RN, CRNP

1998 **Restraint-Free Care: Individualized Approaches for Frail Elders**

   Neville E. Strumpf, PhD, RN, C, FAAN, Joanne Patterson Robinson, PhD, RN, Joan S. Wagner, MSN, CRNP, and Lois K. Evans, DNSc, RN, FAAN

1998 **Home Care for Older Adults: A Guide for Families and Other Caregivers—Text and Instructor's Manual/Lesson Plan**

   Mary Ann Rosswurm, EdD, RN, CS, FAAN

D1569607

Mary Ann Rosswurm, EdD, RN, CS, FAAN is currently the director of the Center for Nursing Research at the Camcare Health Education and Research Institute in Charleston, West Virginia. She has worked in the field of aging and health care for more than 25 years as a nurse practitioner, researcher, and educator. Her efforts have focused on improving hospital care, home care, and nursing home care for functionally dependent elderly persons with chronic health problems. She has worked extensively with family caregivers of persons with Alzheimer's disease and strokes. Dr. Rosswurm has collaborated with the contributors of this book in the past. They are well recognized for their expertise in the care of older adults and family caregivers.

Home Care for Older Adults
A Guide for Families and Other Caregivers

Mary Ann Rosswurm
EdD, RN, CS, FAAN
Editor

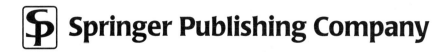 **Springer Publishing Company**

Springer Publishing Company, Inc.
536 Broadway
New York, NY 10012-3955

Cover design by Janet Joachim
Acquisitions Editor: Ruth Chasek
Production Editor: Helen Song

99 00 01 02 / 5 4 3 2

Library of Congress Cataloging-in-Publication Data

Home care for older adults : a guide for families and other caregivers
    / Mary Ann Rosswurm, editor.
        p.   cm.
    Includes index.
    ISBN 0-8261-1231-5
    1. Geriatric nursing.   2. Aged—Home care.   3. Caregivers.
    I. Rosswurm, Mary Ann.
    RC954.H574   1998
    362.1'9897—dc21   98-8674
                                                                      CIP

Printed in the United States of America

Contents

Contributors

Cornelia Beck, PhD, RN, FAAN
Professor and Associate Dean for Research and Evaluation
University of Arkansas for Medical Sciences
College of Nursing
Little Rock, Arkansas

Jane Campbell, MSN, RN, CS
Gerontological Clinical Nurse Specialist
University of North Carolina
Memorial Hospital
Chapel Hill, North Carolina

Brenda Cleary, PhD, RN, CS, FAAN
Executive Director
North Carolina Center for Nursing
Raleigh, North Carolina

Sheila Collier, MNSc, RN
Instructor in Nursing
University of Arkansas for Medical Sciences
College of Nursing
Little Rock, Arkansas

Alicia Curtin, MSN, RN
Gerontological Nurse Practitioner
Clinical Teaching Associate, Family Medicine Residency Program
Brown University School of Medicine
Providence, Rhode Island

Patricia Edwards, MSN, RN
Instructor in Nursing
University of Arkansas Medical Sciences
College of Nursing
Little Rock, Arkansas

Evelyn Fitzwater, DSN, RN, CS
Associate Professor of Clinical Nursing
University of Cincinnati
College of Nursing and Health
Cincinnati, Ohio

Ann Schmidt Luggen, PhD, RN, CS
Professor of Nursing
Northern Kentucky University
Highland Heights, Kentucky

Ann McCracken, PhD, RNC
Professor of Nursing
University of Cincinnati
College of Nursing and Health
Cincinnati, Ohio

Mary Ann Matteson, PhD, RN, CS, FAAN
Professor at the University of Texas Health Science Center
San Antonio School of Nursing
San Antonio, Texas

Susan Sherman, MSN, RN
Gerontological Clinical Nurse Specialist
Rex Healthcare
Raleigh, North Carolina

Foreword

Without question, family caregivers are the nation's greatest asset for providing care to older adults. Dramatic changes in the makeup of our population create challenges for the 21st century. Predictions are that, between now and the year 2050, the elderly population will more than double. As many as one in five Americans will be older than age 65 years. The rapid growth of elderly persons older than age 85 years means that increasing numbers of families will have to care for very old, frail relatives. Fewer family caregivers will be available or prepared to care for this increasingly older population. More home care nurses and aides will be needed to assist family caregivers with the care.

In the days of a more rural America, most children experienced caring for older relatives in the home as a normal part of family life. Passing on the value of family caregiving, along with caregiving knowledge and skills, was part of the custom. In today's mobile society, fewer adults have the opportunity to learn from such family caregiving experiences. At the same time, caregiving challenges are greater with more women employed, smaller families, and sicker older adults recovering from illnesses at home rather than in the hospital. Even without adequate training and skills, family caregivers are expected to provide the bulk of care and to know how to find and use existing services.

Caregiver burden is well described by families caring for older members with dementia and with chronic physical illnesses. The many stresses of caregiving often result in poor health and a lower quality of life for both caregiver and care recipient. Given that community-based care is the watchword for the 21st century, and that family caregivers provide the bulk of community care, we need to support family caregiving. We need more attention to caregiver knowledge and skills regarding care management as well as methods of stress reduction.

Home Care for Older Adults: A Guide for Families and Other Caregivers goes a long way to correct the gaps in information currently available to families and to home care aides and nurses working with the family caregivers. It is rooted in the framework of *learned resourcefulness*, emphasizing health promotion as an achievable outcome of the caregiving experience. The content of the book emphasizes aspects of the caregiving experience that are often most troubling for those called on to provide the care. It acknowledges caregiving as a part of the life cycle. *Home Care for Older Adults: A Guide for Families and Other Caregivers* will increase caregiver knowledge, skills, and motivation, helping to strengthen a resource invaluable for meeting the needs of an aging nation.

LOIS K. EVANS, DNSc, RN, FAAN
Professor and Viola MacInnes/Independence Chair in Nursing
University of Pennsylvania School of Nursing
Philadelphia, Pennsylvania

Acknowledgments

Many people contributed to this book. I am grateful to the family caregivers and older adults who shared their life experiences and demonstrated the strength of the human spirit. They have taught me much.

I appreciated the opportunity to work on this book with an outstanding group of nurse colleagues, whose specialized knowledge of aging and home care helped to make this book a valuable resource.

Throughout the editing process and many typing revisions, I was fortunate to have the expert secretarial assistance of Pam Williams, Inga Trout, and Angela Stroupe.

Barbara McCallum was there when I needed her to read and critique the first edited draft of the book. She was conscientious and committed to her assignment.

Bonnie Pfohl spent many hours discussing the chapter themes with me, so she could capture the intended feelings and thoughts with her drawings. Her original artwork appears throughout the book.

I am most grateful to Richard Rosswurm, my husband, who supported my working on this project over months of weekends. He assisted with the editing, critiqued the book from a layperson's perspective, and made invaluable suggestions.

MARY ANN ROSSWURM

1

Introduction to Caregiving

Mary Ann Rosswurm

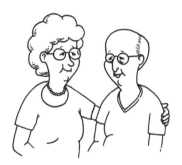
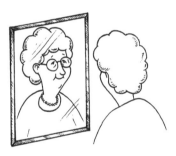

INTRODUCTION TO CAREGIVING

Did you ever think you would be the caregiver for an aging parent, a spouse, or maybe both? Do you feel unprepared, uncertain, or over-whelmed about becoming a caregiver? You are not alone with your feelings. Today thousands of family caregivers are giving more care to frail elderly persons than at any other time. The demand for fam-ily caregivers and other home caregivers will become even greater as the elderly population continues to grow larger and older.

Changes in the family structure and in the health care and work environments make caregiving more difficult. Although both women and men are involved in caregiving, most family caregivers are elderly or middle-aged women, usually wives or adult daughters. The care receiver is typically an older adult with two or more chronic health problems, which limit ability to carry out daily functions. These limitations in basic functional ability are often permanent and require ongoing assistance from a caregiver. Caring for an older person who is functionally dependent becomes even more stressful if the dependent person also has memory loss and behavioral problems.

Most dependent older adults need *caring* rather than high-tech *curing*. Caring focuses on promoting comfort, preventing complications, and maintaining quality of life. Although all caregivers cope with similar problems, each caregiver situation is unique. The caregiver situation is affected by such factors as the general condition of the person needing care, the amount and length of time needed for caregiving, and the health and resources of the caregiver. Other elements that affect caregiving are the nature of the relationship between the caregiver and care recipient, the cultural beliefs about family caregiving, and the support available from friends, family members, and the community.

Caregiving can certainly be a positive and rewarding experience, but it can also create daily struggles with conflicting emotions and strains on energy and health. Caregivers may experience a sense of hopelessness and lack of control as they are faced with an increasing number of losses and demands. Not having things the "way they used to be" and the uncertainty of the future create a great deal of stress.

OVERVIEW OF THE CAREGIVING GUIDE

The goal of this book is to help you to become a resourceful caregiver. A resourceful caregiver is one who copes with the changing demands of caregiving by using objective information for solving problems and planning care. A resourceful caregiver is aware of the importance of self-care and getting support and additional resources when needed. Although this book was written primarily for the family caregiver, the information is also important for other caregivers who work closely with the family caregivers.

There are three main steps for becoming a resourceful caregiver.

- Think positive thoughts
- Get information
- Seek reinforcement

Each chapter in this caregiver book is divided into sections on these steps. The information is not focused on a particular disease, but on the most common problems that caregivers experience as they care for older persons with impaired physical or mental functions.

"Gran" presents the information in a way that helps you to become a resourceful caregiver (see Figure 1.1). Gran serves as your teacher and guide. She brings together the knowledge, experience, and research findings of health professionals, particularly nurses who specialize in the care of older adults (geriatrics or gerontology). Gran also shares practical tips gained from family caregivers who have cared for a dependent or frail older adult at home.

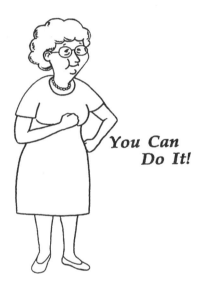

You Can Do It!

Gran presents important information about caregiving in an easy-to-read way. Follow her throughout the book, and you will feel better prepared and confident about caregiving. You can learn more about caregiving by reading this book on your own or as part of a caregiver training program in your community. In a group training program, you can learn new information with guidance and feedback from a nurse instructor. You can also exchange ideas with other caregivers. You need to explore what type of training is available in your community and decide what method of learning works best for you. You are off to a good start by the fact that you are reading this book and trying to get more information about caregiving.

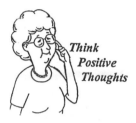

Think
Positive
Thoughts

In each chapter, an icon or symbol of Gran appears at the beginning of the three main chapter sections, reminding you of these steps of resourceful caregiving. In the first section, you see Gran encouraging you to think positive thoughts and to get rid of any negative messages that you may be giving yourself. Negative messages interfere with your ability to think clearly and gain new information for solving caregiving problems. The content in this section of the chapter might include an inspiring case story, a quotation, or some positive self-statements (affirmations), such as, "I can handle difficult situations"; "I can take one thing at a time"; or "I know how to seek help when it is needed."

You are encouraged to think positive thoughts and do some relaxation exercises to prepare you to take in new information and solve problems. The following are some examples of relaxation exercises that you might try before reading the chapter or dealing with a stressful caregiving situation.

Deep Breathing

- Sit upright in a comfortable position.
- Keep your back straight and feet flat.
- Place hands on your abdomen or stomach area.
- Inhale slowly, counting to five, pretending your mouth is around a straw.
- Feel your abdomen expand.
- Hold your breath for two counts.
- Exhale slowly through the pretend straw, counting to 10 as you exhale.

Shoulder Relaxation

- Shrug both shoulders upward toward your ears.
- Tighten shoulders together, and hold for 10 counts.
- Move shoulders back and around.
- Relax.

Also, research on *humor* has shown that a daily diet of smiles and laughs helps to keep the mind, body, and spirit healthy. You are encouraged to look on the lighter side and laugh whenever you can.

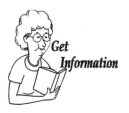

Get Information

In the next main section of each chapter, Gran helps you "get information" about specific caregiving problems. Most caregiving problems are connected to the basic activities of daily living (ADLs). These activities include eating, getting in and out of bed, walking, dressing, bathing and grooming, and toileting and bowel and bladder (continence) care. Dependent or frail older adults often need assistance from the caregiver with one or more of these ADLs. Health complications that lead to hospitalization or nursing home admission often occur when these basic needs are not met. No matter what the chronic illness or disability, the caregiver deals with problems involved in these basic needs.

Other chapters in the book provide information about aspects of caregiving that present special challenges. These topics include attending to self-care of the caregiver, communicating with the person receiving care and with health professionals, managing confusion and behavior problems, and coping with loss and death.

Gran presents the information in a way that will prepare you to use problem-solving skills as you manage the common problems of caregiving. You will be able to identify problems by learning which changes are normal aging changes and which are abnormal symptoms that need to be reported. You will be prepared to communicate with the physician, nurse, and other health professionals to set realistic goals and to develop the best plan of care.

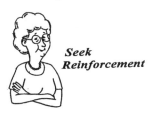

Seek Reinforcement

In the last main section of each chapter, Gran gives you the message to seek reinforcement. You are encouraged to give yourself daily rewards for achieving goals. You are also given information about when and where to get additional help and reinforcement. This section may also include review questions and exercises to help you evaluate how well you learned the new information and skills. By getting positive feedback, you gain confidence in your ability to cope with difficult situations. If you are in a caregiver training group, you can also discuss different strategies for specific problems.

The caregiver's role has rewards and strains. Both the caregiver and care receiver need to gain some sense of control over the sometimes uncontrollable circumstances and changes. As you become a more resourceful caregiver, you will learn to keep feelings and responsibilities in balance and adapt to the demands of your caregiving situation. Resourceful caregiving requires that the family caregiver and home health aide know the limits of their personal resources and seek reinforcement from others.

As Gran says, "You can do it," if you know how and when and where to get help. Read the next chapter carefully. It stresses the importance of self-care as an essential ingredient for effective caregiving.

2

Self-Care of the Caregiver

Evelyn Fitzwater

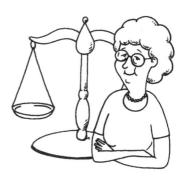

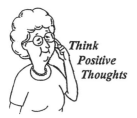

Think Positive Thoughts

As human beings, we are composed of body, mind, and spirit. We most often think of "body care" when we talk about taking care of ourselves and other people. Our first concern, of necessity, is to make sure we get enough food, water, and shelter. Then, we may consider factors that may be important to keep our minds healthy, such as being stimulated by reading, studying, thinking, or meditation. Our emotions and feelings are recognized as part of who we are, and we work on keeping emotional balance. In addition, we have a spiritual aspect of our lives that keeps us connected to nature, the things that we see, and also the things we are unable to see yet believe in. Most of us spend each day trying to balance the needs of our body, mind, and spirit. Depending on many factors, we may be more or less successful on any given day. It is not surprising when we find ourselves taking on more responsibility, such as caregiving, that the balancing act gets a little tougher.

As a caregiver you are a special resource. You are helping another person to meet the everyday needs that all human beings have. Caregiving is one way to gain personal satisfaction in physical work for the body, problem solving for the mind, and the feeling of being needed and appreciated for the spirit. But you need to understand that the caregiving role is only one aspect of who you are and what you do. It is easy to become so involved in the caregiving of others that you forget to take care of yourself. You have only one turn in this experience called life, and you deserve to live it—not just to survive. You can be a *resourceful* caregiver and continue to have a life apart from the caregiver role if you remember to maintain *balance:*

B *Be realistic* about what you can expect from yourself (be gentle with yourself).

A *Ask for help* when you need it (from family, friends, or outside agencies).

L *Listen* to your body, mind, and spirit for signs of exhaustion, confusion, anger, frustration, and emptiness.

A *Allow* your care recipient to do something for you or give something to you (someone who is "taking" needs to "give back" for their own balance as well).

N *Network* with others for information (natural networks, such as church, synagogue, community, support groups, and health care professionals).

C *Care* as much for yourself as you care for others (if you are half full, how can you give at full speed?).

E *Enjoy* a laugh, or further develop your sense of humor (you will not get out of this life alive, so you might as well take life and yourself a little less seriously!).

THE CAREGIVER AND SELF-CARE

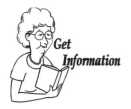

Get Information

"We are family. I have all my sisters with me." The words of this rock song may drift through the minds of the many family caregivers, 75% of whom are women, usually wives, adult daughters, or daughters-in-law. Caregiving usually involves women, and the expectation is that they are the ones who will fulfill the roles of caregiver and nurturer because "it's always been that way." Most women caregivers of older adults are also parenting their own children. Although men make up a much smaller percentage of caregivers, all husbands, sons, and brothers are also affected by the caregiving process in some way.

Most caregiver time is spent in providing daily personal care to an older adult experiencing a chronic illness. A significant amount of the caregiver role is assisting with basic daily activities, such as mobility, eating, dressing, toileting, transferring, and bathing. The caregiver also helps with other daily tasks important to the care recipient's well-being including answering and placing telephone calls, using transportation, managing medicines and money, shopping, doing laundry, and maintaining the home. The caregiver may be faced with caring for a person who is mentally impaired as a result of dementia. In this case, the caregiver copes with the loss of a relationship and with communication problems.

As a caregiver you have tremendous responsibilities. Not only are you giving the care recipient personal care, but you may also need to handle medical aspects of care. If you have no training in health care, these responsibilities could be overwhelming. In many instances, you may be performing care that would take three different shifts of staff to provide in a nursing facility or hospital. In addition to your caregiving responsibilities, you are also maintaining many other roles.

Self-care, the C in *balance*, becomes vital if you are to keep up your energy level. Maintaining wellness of your body, mind, and spirit is as important as anything you do for someone else. If you consider yourself an important part of someone else's life, think of the possible effect of neglecting to take care of yourself as much as you think of the caring for someone else. Make your health and wellness a priority.

FOCUS ON KEEPING YOURSELF WELL

Be mindful that you need to eat a balanced diet, get enough rest and sleep, exercise, and enjoy some leisure time every day. If you skip meals, drink caffeine or alcohol to excess, eat on the run, or eat a high-fat, sugary diet, you will find your energy at a low level. You need to get enough rest so that you are refreshed and able to function well each day. Sleep allows the body and mind to get ready for another day. If your sleep is routinely disturbed, you may need to consult your physician or nurse for help. You need adequate rest and sleep to be the best you can for yourself and others. Regular exercise helps manage stress, keeps your body fit, keeps your mind relaxed, and lifts your spirits. Leisure activities are also important in keeping well. You need a time out. You will find that you are more able to cope with life in general if you allow yourself time to do things that you enjoy.

Remember to schedule your check-ups for medical and dental care so that you are promoting your health and attempting to prevent illness. Be aware that if you neglect your own health, you risk the possibility that you may become ill yourself and may not be able to provide the needed care.

"Everybody needs somebody sometime." These words of an old song express perfectly the human need for social contact. People need people in their lives to share conversation, enjoyment, and relaxation. Although the demands of caregiving may reduce the time you have to spend with friends and family, take time out to spend with others. If you eliminate the social aspects of your life, you may feel isolated and resentful about the caregiving situation. Family caregivers usually need assistance with caregiving to have some time for social activities.

MANAGING STRESS

Although a certain amount of stress is needed in life, you do not want it to get out of control. Here are some tips to help keep stress in balance.

- Prepare for the morning the night before. Make lunches, lay out clothes, etc.

- Do not rely exclusively on your memory. Write down only points you want to remember. Have duplicate keys made. Stress plays tricks on memory.
- Plan ahead, and avoid putting off doing things that need to be done.
- Have realistic goals and expectations. Do not try to be a perfectionist.
- Ask questions, and ask for repeat directions (if needed). Ask what others expect of you, and be clear about what you are capable of doing.
- Learn to say no. You can do only so much.
- Unplug your telephone once in a while, or let the answering machine take a message.
- Take a "time out."
- Treat yourself to a relaxing bath, meditate, or read without being interrupted.
- Remember to *breathe*. Take several deep, breaths before, during, and after stressful situations or anytime.
- Be gentle with yourself. Remember, you are a helper, not a magician.
- Remind yourself that you cannot change people or certain situations, but you can change how you respond to them.

LAUGHTER IS THE BEST MEDICINE

Laughter has many positive affects. Laughter is useful in releasing tension, reducing pain, improving breathing, and generally improving your mood while lifting your spirits. If you lose your sense of humor, you lose your perspective on life. Accept the importance of laughing at yourself and being able to laugh about situations.

Try a few time-tested techniques for increasing humor and laughter in your life. Read the comics, funny books, or jokes. Listen to tapes of comedians or old radio shows. Watch humorous movies or videos. Share a laugh with the person for whom you are caring. Try to go to social events where there is a lot of fun and joy. Smile, laugh, and enjoy.

If you experience a change in your sense of humor or laughter has gone out of your life, you may need to talk about what is going on in your life with a friend or someone else you trust. Perhaps you may need to consider talking to a counselor, if you are feeling hopelessness or continued sadness along with a loss of your sense of humor.

THE CAREGIVER'S BILL OF RIGHTS

Did you know that caregivers have rights? Because you are caring for another, you do not automatically give up your basic rights to life, liberty, and the pursuit of happiness. The following statements are taken from the *Caregiver's Handbook* by Mike Moldeven.

Caregivers have the right to

- Appropriate training in caregiving along with accurate, understandable information about the condition and needs of the care recipient.
- Appreciation and emotional support for their decision to accept the challenge of providing care.
- Protection of their assets and financial future without severing their relationship with the care receiver.
- Respite care during emergencies and in order to care for their own health, spirit, and relationships.
- Help from all family members, both men and women in the care for aging relatives.
- Provide care at home as long as physically, financially, and emotionally feasible; however, when it is no longer feasible, caregivers have the obligation to explore other alternatives, such as a residential care facility.
- Professional care that recognizes the importance of comfort and the concerns of older people and caregivers.

These are rights, insofar as possible, of those who care for others. Some of the caregiver rights may appear to be common sense in action, but many caregivers believe that they give up their individual right to a life when they agree to care for another. If you read down the list of rights, you will notice that observing the rights of the care-giver will help ensure that the person receiving care will have needs met. A successful relationship between caregiver and care receiver is one in which both people feel valued and respected. It takes some trial and error to reach a balance in the caregiving relationship. You have the right to be less than perfect and so does your care receiver. Give yourself some positive self-talk when times get rough, and re-member to ask for help when you need it. Family members often will say, "Nobody can take care of him or her like I can." This is probably true. But a worn-out, burned-out you cannot care for an-other unless you take care of yourself. Caregivers need to be aware that one person's rights should not cancel the rights of another to pursue a fulfilling life, be free to make choices, and find happiness. As a caregiver, you deserve no less in life.

IMPACT OF CAREGIVING AND FAMILY RELATIONSHIPS

Each family is unique and experiences life differently. Family mem-bers have a unique history with each other. Some families experience positive outcomes from caregiving for an elderly family member with a chronic illness. For example, some people slow down their lives and appreciate the temporary nature of life, valuing their time together. Instead of growing apart and being resentful, family mem-bers can grow closer and more tolerant of one another. Caring for an older person with chronic illness inevitably changes roles and the way things used to be. Success in meeting the challenges presented by caregiving includes *grieving* the losses that come with these changes and establishing new balances of personal and family re-sources. The care recipient, family caregiver, and other caregivers may express their grief in different ways. Common reactions in-clude feelings of anger, guilt, and depression.

In addition to grief, a healthy dose of guilt may be the order of the day. "Guilt is the gift that keeps on giving." This saying is espe-cially true when you are faced with the struggle between your feel-ings as an independent person and as a caregiver for someone who is depending on you. You may feel trapped in the situation and then feel bad that you feel trapped. You may remember experiencing hurts from your loved one, feel anger, and then feel guilty because you felt anger at the one who now is suffering such loss. You may wish you were not involved in caregiving for any number of reasons and experience guilt as a result. You may lose control and speak harshly to relatives that you perceive as not pitching in to help or not being supportive of your caregiving efforts and then feel guilty. You may also feel guilty about being angry about the role reversal, which has you "parenting" a parent or spouse.

Do we give out of obligation or love? If we give out of a sense of duty, without love, we feel guilty. Family members often say that "it is my duty" to do this, or I have an obligation to do that for my relative. Family members often ask: "If we give out of a sense of obligation, is that OK?" Many family members find themselves pressured into being the primary caregiver because they live closer to or with the person in need of care, or everyone else in the family works. In situations where family members have taken on the caregiving responsibility through pressure, there is enough guilt to go around for everyone.

To break the cycle, a family conference might be in order. But many families have no knowledge about how to talk with each other and do problem solving together. If a family conference is not a method your family is familiar with, consult your physician or nurse about getting a referral for assistance.

Family members often experience some common reactions when faced with caregiving responsibilities and challenges. Some members will deny the seriousness of the situation they face and act as though nothing has changed. These members need to be assisted to understand the realities of the situation and how they can help their relative. Other family members may become too involved with the care receiver and complete even the slightest task for the person. This reactive behavior serves only to increase dependency and may lead to frustration, anger, and depression for both caregiver and care receiver. The caregiver needs to be made aware of this negative behavior and maintain balance.

Anger may be a response to any situation of change. As a rule, we do not readily accept change that did not involve our input. Unrelieved anger has a way of erupting unexpectedly. We may inappropriately take out feelings of anger and frustration on someone else. For example, an angry caregiver may shout, verbally or physically abuse, or humiliate the person receiving the care. This behavior is clearly inappropriate and may bring on guilt for the caregiver and loss of self-esteem for the care receiver. Anger can be diffused by admitting feeling angry, talking to someone about the problems that are at the root of the anger, and planning to take action to get rid of the anger. Some helpful strategies include getting involved in a support group to talk with people who have had similar experiences and engaging in physical exercise, deep breathing, and meditation.

Family members report that they sometimes experience spiritual distress when they are faced with the multiple responsibilities of caregiving. This spiritual distress often accompanies feelings of hopelessness and powerlessness. Sometimes people report a loss of faith in God and blame God for their situation. Many times they ask questions like: "Why me?"; "Why is this happening to my family?"; or "Why won't God lift this burden?" Sometimes spiritual distress leads to a sense of having no purpose in life or no connection to others. People who struggle with change and loss often draw on their spiritual beliefs to help them cope. These people will benefit from support and reinforcement of their beliefs.

HOW TO FIND AND GET HELP

As a family caregiver, you expect a lot from yourself. Be realistic about what you can hope to accomplish on your own and what you can and should reasonably expect from others. Caregivers often have many roles. When a family caregiving role is added on top of all the existing roles, it can become overwhelming. Many times caregiving is cut short by illness or burn-out as a result of caregivers thinking they could do it all. The situation may become so stressful that the caregiver and family finally give up and take the care receiver to the emergency room or nursing home without considering alternatives, perhaps because they are not aware of what services are available or how to access them. Family caregivers need to work closely with other home caregivers.

Before you begin to explore formal community services, you will need to get organized and pull together information. It is most helpful if you have answers at your fingertips so that you can assist in providing an overview and specifics to the agency at the time you speak to them. You will need to include a medical file (doctor's diagnoses), medication list, and medical emergency plan. A financial file should list bank accounts, financial advisors, income statement, and monthly expense statement. The health insurance file needs to include any and all policies and payers. A bills and receipts file is helpful for ready reference or price comparison. A legal documents file is essential; a copy of the person's will and medical power of attorney should be kept here.

After you have gathered and organized the information suggested previously, it is important to have a clear idea of what kind of help is needed. Your physician can be an excellent source of referral for services. You can also contact a geriatric assessment center that provides comprehensive health services to older adults. The geriatric assessment center can be an outpatient ambulatory clinic or hospital-based, inpatient service. Usually, a geriatric physician, a doctor who specialized in care of the older adult, will provide the medical services. The physician may work with a team of specialists in the care of older adults, such as a nurse, social worker, and dietitian. They can perform a comprehensive examination that includes physical, emotional, social, and financial assessment. Following the assessment, the team offers suggestions and makes referrals to helping agencies in the community. Hospitals in your area may be able to help you find a geriatric assessment center or other health care professionals who specialize in the care of older people.

The following list includes several examples of support services for caregivers which you may find helpful as resources. These services are only examples of services and are not meant to represent all available community services.

- *Respite care*—temporary help for caregivers (2 hrs a day–2 weeks)
- *Home health care*—nurses, aides, personal care
- *Homemaker*—shopping, laundry, cleaning, cooking, etc.
- *Meals-on-Wheels*—home delivered meals
- *Transportation*—doctor visits, shopping, etc.
- *Handyperson*—repairs, lawncare, etc.

- *Friendly visitor*—home social visits
- *Adult day care*—physical, emotional, social care center
- *Geriatric care manager*—nurse, social worker coordinates care
- *Telecare*—daily telephone reassurance
- *Caregiver support group*—informal discussion group for caregivers

Community services can be located for you by your state Office on Aging, Area Agencies on Aging, local senior centers, your physician's office, the American Association of Retired Persons (AARP), your employer human resources office, and friends or acquaintances.

There are also many informal services available to caregivers through such organizations as churches, synagogues, volunteer agencies, and social clubs. Remember, balance means having the courage to receive as well as to give and remembering that taking care of yourself is a healthy thing to do.

THE NURSING HOME DECISION

The words "nursing home" often bring unpleasant thoughts and feelings to many families who are caring for older adults. All nursing homes are frequently stereotyped as the places where older people are warehoused, neglected, or even mistreated. This viewpoint often makes the decision about choosing a nursing home more difficult because of the fear and guilt it produces in the family. A nursing home may be the appropriate treatment option, but because of negative feelings, the nursing home decision is viewed as a last resort. You may have heard stories about how some parents have asked their children to promise "never to put me in a nursing home." The very idea of entering a nursing home may seem like getting a death sentence to some people. Be aware that there are some wonderful nursing homes, where people get the skilled care they need, and families are able to meet their needs as well.

The decision to use nursing home care is often painful; however, sometimes nursing home care may be the needed level of care. Sometimes giving people what they need, rather than what they or we want, is the best way to show our love.

At times family members will disagree among themselves about where and how the caregiving should be done for your relative. The stressful situation may result in family arguments and hurt feelings. A family conference with a professional (e.g., doctor, nurse, social worker, counselor, or clergy) may be helpful.

One way of dealing with negative feelings about nursing homes is to learn everything you can about nursing homes before the need for making the decision. Information will help reduce the fear and guilt often experienced when thinking about a nursing home. You can begin to learn about nursing home care by talking to friends or acquaintances who have experience with nursing homes. Get information from your local Area Agency on Aging, hospital social workers, physicians, nurses, and the health department. Before deciding on nursing home care, you will need to understand the types of nursing homes available, the finances involved, family responsibility, and ways to judge the quality of care provided by a nursing home. Visit several nursing homes, interview staff members, look around, talk to some of the residents, notice the level of cleanliness, the presence of unpleasant odors, and the general atmosphere.

Remember to be realistic and understand that there is no perfect nursing home. However, there are many nursing facilities that provide various levels of homelike care. Nursing homes can provide the needed care. Exercising the option to use the nursing home in place of family caregivers is not an easy decision to make but sometimes is the only practical decision. Trust your instincts.

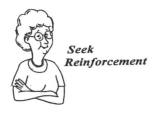

Seek Reinforcement

Caregiving for a dependent older adult can bring experiences that challenge the body, mind, and spirit balance of all those who are involved. Caregivers need to be aware that the challenges can be met if you are willing to use the strategies found in this guide. These strategies have proved helpful in the caregiving situation. You need to be aware of your feelings and those of others about what is happening. Develop positive attitudes about the experience by keeping it in perspective. Take advantage of help available from family, friends, and community resources. Be willing to make decisions, and take actions that help you keep a healthy balance in your life. Superman is a myth, and Superwoman does not exist. Remember, the best you can do *is* the best you can do.

ADDITIONAL READING SUGGESTIONS

Beattie, M. (1990). *The language of letting go: Daily meditations for code-pendents.* New York: Harper Collins.

Caring for the caregiver: A guide for living with Alzheimer's disease. (1994). Sponsored by Parke-Davis. Morris Plains, NJ: Warner-Lambert.

Greenberg, V. (1995). *Children of a certain age.* San Francisco: Jossey-Bass.

Manning, D. (1987). *When loves gets tough: The nursing home decision.* Hereford, TX: In-Sight Books.

Schaef, A. W. (1990). *Meditations for women who do too much.* San Francisco: Harper Collins.

Schaef, A. W. (1996). *Meditations for people who (may) worry too much.* New York: Ballantine Books.

INTERNET RESOURCES

http//.angelfire.com/tn/nursing home/index.html
http//.www.Caregiver911.com/html/ask_dr_caregiver.html
http//.www.caregivers911.com.html/resources
http//www.geocites.com/Hotsprings/2021
http//www.examiner.com Link: The Caregivers

3

Communication

Brenda Cleary and Mary Ann Matteson

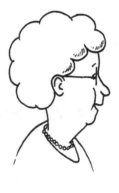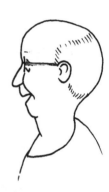

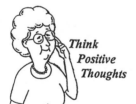

Think Positive Thoughts

Good communication is extremely important to healthy relationships but is usually an ongoing challenge for most of us. Breakdown in communication is a rather common occurrence among family members who are providing care for a dependent family member. Role changes, fatigue, stress, and depression can alter the way we communicate. The good news is that there are some techniques and strategies you can learn to improve communication. It is usually the way we say things that can make a difference. As a caregiver, it is also useful to learn some strategies for communicating better with health care professionals, such as doctors and nurses. You can do that, too!

Communication is also influenced by aging changes in vision and hearing as well as by the sensory diseases. As people age, there are almost always changes in vision and hearing. Most likely, the person you care for (as well as perhaps you, yourself) needs eyeglasses and may not hear quite as well as in the past. The good news is that most people adapt very well to these changes with some simple modifications.

AGING CHANGES IN VISION AND HEARING

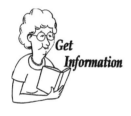

Get Information

In the information section that follows, I will describe common age-related changes in vision and hearing and how to deal with them. I will also talk about how to recognize symptoms of more serious disorders of the eyes. First, review this information about age-related changes. The following are facts about vision in later life:

- Almost half of all cases of legal blindness occur in persons aged 65 years or older.
- Farsightedness, resulting in being unable to see close objects clearly, is most common.
- We become less sensitive to light but more sensitive to glare with age.
- It becomes more difficult to adjust when going from lighted to darkened areas.
- Vision becomes less sharp in general.
- Colors, particularly darker colors, become less clear because of yellowing of the eye's lens.
- The ability to judge depth and height decreases.
- There may be a decline of peripheral vision, that is, a narrowing of the field of vision.
- Visual problems can make it more difficult to care for oneself.

Problem-solving strategies for maximizing vision include using bright lighting; color contrast; visual aids, such as eyeglasses and magnifying lenses; and large-print reading materials. From a safety standpoint, it is important to allow time to adapt to changes in lighting. Night lights are also recommended at bedtime. If the person you are caring for is having trouble with peripheral vision (seeing off to the sides), it is good to take extra care to position food or other objects within the field of vision.

DISORDERS OF THE EYE

The commonest diseases or disorders of the eyes in later life include cataracts, glaucoma, macular degeneration, and diabetic retinopathy. Regular eye examinations are important for early diagnosis and treatment of these eye problems.

CATARACTS

Cataracts occur when the lens of the eye becomes cloudy, resulting in a gradual loss of vision in one or both eyes. Cataracts cause increasing problems with glare, a darkening of the vision, and a loss of sharpness. Treatment of this disorder involves removing the cataracts and replacing the lens or correcting the vision with contacts or eyeglasses.

GLAUCOMA

Glaucoma occurs when the pressure inside the eye increases. Such pressure can cause damage to the nerves inside the eye and blindness if not treated. Treatment most commonly involves the use of eye drops to decrease the pressure within the eye.

MACULAR DEGENERATION

Macular degeneration involves damage to the macula, which is the most important part of the eye located on the retina. Unfortunately, most cases of macular degeneration are not treatable, although some cases have improved with laser treatments.

DIABETIC RETINOPATHY

Diabetic retinopathy occurs when the blood supply to the retina inside the eye is decreased because of blood vessel changes brought on by diabetes. The best treatment for this kind of eye condition is prevention—in other words, keeping diabetes under control so that there is less damage to the blood vessel as a complication of diabetes, although laser treatment and surgery may also be used for this condition.

HEARING IN LATER LIFE

Problems with hearing usually increase the older we get, with more than 40% of people older than age 75 years having hearing problems. Most commonly, older people have trouble hearing high-pitched sounds. A buildup of ear wax can greatly interfere with hearing. Certain medicines can also affect hearing. Hearing loss can result in social isolation.

It is a good idea to have ears checked during a physical. If there is any buildup of earwax, the problem can easily be corrected by irrigating the ears. Another simple but effective technique in caring for someone with a hearing loss is to face the person directly and to speak very slowly and clearly. Always get the person's attention before you speak. Use gestures as you are talking. Keep the background noise down and try to resist the temptation to shout to make the person hear. Try lowering the pitch of your voice.

Hearing evaluations may determine that a hearing aid is needed to improve hearing. The following guidelines should be helpful for hearing aid users:

- Practice inserting and removing the hearing aid until you can do these things easily. Get help if you have questions.
- Wear the hearing aid 4 to 5 hours at first. After a week, it should be worn all day.
- Remove the hearing aid before going to bed, bathing, or showering.
- Make sure the battery is inserted correctly. Follow + sign for placement of + side of battery. If there is no on-off switch, open

the battery case at night to shut the aid off; this will conserve the battery power. If there is an M-T-O (microphone-telephone-off) switch on the aid, turn to *O* for off at night. Don't forget to turn back to *M* in the morning to turn the aid on. Store unused batteries in a cool, dry, place.

- Clean the ear mold daily with a damp cloth. Once a week wipe the mold with a cloth dampened with mild soapy water. Do not immerse the mold in water. If the ear mold gets plugged with wax, clean it out with toothpick or bent paper clip or wax-removing tool—carefully!

- Change the batteries every 10 days to 2 weeks. If a whistle (feedback) is *not* there when the volume control is fully on, change the battery. If no whistle is heard despite a new battery, then the problem is in the aid itself.

Remember that the aid is a mechanical instrument. Sounds and voices are made louder, not clearer. Expectations should be realistic. The extra noise may annoy you at first, but in a short time you will get used to hearing background sounds. If you have problems, have the audiologist or hearing aid dealer check the hearing aid.

RESOURCEFUL COMMUNICATION
AMONG FAMILY MEMBERS

Kind words can be short and easy to speak, but their echoes are truly endless.

—Mother Teresa

Remember that communication is bound to be affected by changes in roles. Research has shown that there may be some strain associated with the caregiving role as well as the role of receiving care. Spouses, who represent about half of all family caregivers, have to make some special adjustments along with their mates. A spouse who provides care may have to take on additional responsibilities previously taken care of by the ill partner. Intimacy may be affected by giving and receiving very personal care. Also, both the caregiver and the care receiver may be fatigued.

Providing care for a parent often creates distress in terms of a "role reversal," that is, providing care for someone who has in the past been the provider of care. A grieving process is associated with changes in roles. At the same time, a special bond can develop in a caregiving situation. A new and different kind of closeness may result, and there are definite rewards associated with caregiving.

Talk about the changes you are experiencing (together or to someone else who is a good listener). Try to create situations where it feels more like old times; for example, capitalize on the remaining strengths of the person receiving care. Find activities you can still do and enjoy together; reminisce. Do something special for yourself (to make you feel like your old self). Seek support from other family members, friends, health professionals, churches, and other community organizations and support groups in your area.

Stress, in general, can hinder communication. Some of the commonest causes of stress in the caregiving situation stem from personal concerns and worries about relationships with others. Personal concerns may include worry about your health and finances. You may also be concerned because you are finding it difficult to perform the caregiving tasks. Because of the little time you have for yourself, you may feel resentment or guilt. Problems or concerns about your relationships with family and friends may arise when you feel others don't understand or don't care enough to call or visit.

When your stress and personal concerns begin to increase, take time out to talk about the situation. Recognize and discuss the sometimes overwhelming role of caregiving. Arrange for family meetings and talk about how others can help. Evaluate your relationship with the person for whom you are providing care. Develop a hopeful but realistic sense of the future. Plan for outside social contacts and set aside time for yourself. Recognize when you might be reaching your "wit's end," and seek the help of your physician or nurse.

Pain in either the caregiver or care receiver is another factor that can alter communications. Responses to pain are explained in detail in Chapter 5. People can become withdrawn or depressed when pain is not managed well, and communication decreases.

COMMUNICATING WELL

Effective communication begins with good listening skills. Try to find a quiet place where you won't have constant interruptions or distractions. Most of us find it difficult to listen without, at the same time, thinking about what we will say next. Listen carefully for the meaning the words are trying to convey. Also consider tone of voice, facial expressions, and gestures. Active listening not only involves clearing our own minds, but also checking with the other person to see if you really understood what he or she was trying to say.

Clear, assertive, constructive communication is most likely to occur when you use "I" messages. For example, if the person for whom you are caring has been complaining all day, you might respond: "I know you are uncomfortable, but I feel very frustrated" as opposed to "You are a constant complainer, and you are getting on my nerves!"

Speak slowly and deliberately, in a calm voice. Be aware of your own nonverbal communication and how you can use nonverbal cues to communicate more effectively. Be resourceful in not only getting but giving positive reinforcement. It can work wonders, especially when combined with touching and other forms of affection. Other guidelines for promoting communication, especially involving important matters, include the following:

- Try to hold conversations about serious matters when you both are calm and rested.
- Be open, clear, and calm.
- Keep conversations focused.
- Give the other person a chance to draw conclusions and make choices.
- If the person who is receiving care does not want to talk about something, it is probably best to back off and try again another time.
- End the discussion if either one of you becomes tired or cranky, but leave the door open for future conversations.
- If verbal communication fails, a warm hug may help. Hugs are free, mutually beneficial, and relieve tension.

Sometimes illness itself has profound effects on communication. Dementia not only causes forgetfulness, but often makes it difficult to find the right word. As dementia progresses, the person has difficulty understanding and carrying on any kind of meaningful conversation. Adjustments are necessary as the ability to use speech deteriorates. It becomes important to use simple, familiar words without double meanings and to avoid complex sentences. Give one direction, or ask one question at a time. Use gestures. Allow plenty of time for response and provide reassurance and praise.

An important rule of thumb for communicating with someone experiencing confusion is to avoid arguing. When perceptions of reality differ, arguing only leads to unnecessary frustration.

Strokes almost always affect communication, also resulting in word-finding difficulty. Try to be patient and not critical. Sometimes suggesting a word or offering a visual cue helps. Have the person try writing the message or use gestures to convey the message.

RESOURCEFUL COMMUNICATION
WITH HEALTH CARE PROFESSIONALS

Selecting the right health care professional can be one of the most important decisions you make. Some sources of referrals include family and friends, professional organizations, and consumer groups. Here are some suggested questions to ask about health care professionals.

- Education and experience qualifications of the health professional.
- Cost of services and when payments are due.
- Insurance arrangements.
- Location.
- Hours of operation.
- Ways emergencies are handled.

You will want to evaluate whether the office is clean and well equipped and whether services received are prompt and efficient.

Are examinations thorough? Are you at ease in asking questions, and do you feel that you get thoughtful answers? Are explanations regarding diagnostic findings and treatments clear? Are you provided with options and allowed to make informed choices?

Communication with health professionals is aided by keeping good records at home. Your health records might contain the following information:

- Names, addresses, and telephone numbers of health professionals you see regularly.
- Medical history information.
- List of all prescription and over-the-counter medications.
- Any special treatment instructions.
- Bills and receipts.
- Insurance policy information.

To get the most benefit out of appointments with health care professionals, be organized. Prepare a list of questions. Bring along the appropriate medical histories and lists of medications so that you won't have to carry all these details in your head. When a new medication is prescribed, you will want to obtain the following information:

- What is the medication intended to do?
- Does the medication treat the cause of the problem or only the symptoms?
- When and how should the medication be taken and for how long?
- Are there other medications or foods that interact with this medication?
- What are the side effects?
- How soon will the medication have an effect?
- What should you do if a dose is missed?
- Is there a less expensive generic form of this medication?

Ask for written instructions about tests and treatments. Question what you do not understand. You may need to discuss changes in your health or the condition of the person you are caring for as well as changes in diet, exercise, sleeping patterns, and emotional state.

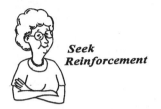

Seek
Reinforcement

Communication involves both listening to understand and speaking to be understood. Your communication will be better if you practice the communication strategies I have presented in this chapter. Think positive thoughts, but do not try to be a superhero in the way you relate to the person receiving your care. Remember that all families have communication breakdowns even in the best of circumstances. Set limits, and do not expect perfection. Do expect conflicting feelings. Remember that the person receiving care may also experience conflicting feelings. However, a positive person keeps things in perspective. Get the information you need and also remember to write down questions for health care professionals. In addition, refer to the resource guide at the end of this book to get further information for special problems.

4

Confusion and Behavior Problems

Mary Ann Rosswurm

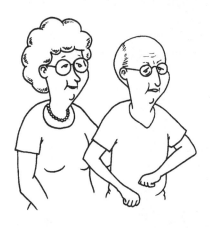

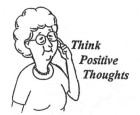

**Think
Positive
Thoughts**

Before you do anything else, take a *deep breath, hold it* for 2 seconds, and *blow it out slowly*. Good! Now close your eyes for a minute, and think about a recent event that brought a smile to your face or made you laugh. If you are having trouble thinking of something, try this: Picture yourself or someone else wearing a big red clown nose. Funny sight, isn't it? Go ahead . . . *laugh out loud*. When things begin getting out of control, laughter helps us to step back and pause for a moment. It gives us a chance to regroup; look at things from a different angle; and think about new ways of managing difficult problems, such as confusion.

Confusion is *not* a normal part of aging. It is caused by disease and medical complications resulting from medications, nutritional problems, injuries, and so forth. Confusion is a condition in which there are serious problems with mental functions (such as attention, memory, and other thinking abilities) as well as inappropriate behaviors. Depending on its cause, confusion can occur suddenly and be treated and reversed. It also can occur gradually and grow progressively worse.

In this chapter, I will be talking about three *D*s that are often associated with confusion. They are *depression, delirium,* and *dementia.* Although the symptoms of these problems can be similar, the causes and treatments are different. Some causes of confusion can be treated and reversed. Other types of confusion become chronic.

Caring for a person with confusion can be stressful for the caregiver. Although researchers and health professionals do not have all the answers to what causes or cures confusion, they have learned much about how to manage confusion and its related problems. Before I discuss that information, let us take a look at some aging changes to see how they can affect cognition or mental functioning.

NORMAL AGING CHANGES AFFECTING MEMORY

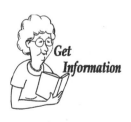

Get Information

Older adults complain about their memories all the time. How often have you heard someone say, "Where did I put my keys?"; "You know, . . . what's his name?"; "Did I tell you this before?"; or "I guess I'm just getting old."

As soon as older adults begin having trouble remembering names or where they left their keys, they think they are getting "senile." Contrary to what many people believe, normal aging does not cause memory loss. Aging may bring some mild *forgetfulness* but not *memory loss.* Becoming anxious or depressed about mild forgetfulness can increase the forgetfulness problem. With age, the brain does lose some cells, but it adapts by increasing the number of connections between cells. Older adults continue to learn and remember new things, although it may take a little more time. In fact, studies show that as you age you can reach higher levels of understanding about the important things of life.

The aging body in general adapts less effectively to stress and is at greater risk for *mechanical, physical,* and *emotional* blocks to memory. You can do many things to prevent or adjust to these blocks before they seriously affect memory and interfere with daily functioning.

MECHANICAL BLOCKS

Memory changes can be understood better by looking at how information gets in and out of the brain. The human brain has four basic memory processes. First, it *takes in* information through the senses (vision, hearing, touch, taste, and smell). Then it *interprets* the information, *stores* it in short-term and then in long-term memory, and finally *retrieves and uses* the information as needed. Normal aging changes in the senses, especially vision and hearing, can create mechanical blocks to memory. If the senses inaccurately pick up information, then inaccurate information will be stored in memory. An older adult may appear "confused," when, in fact, the problem is related to a mechanical block.

Another mechanical block is distraction. Older adults are distracted more easily by background noises, which interfere with attention to the new information. For example, if you are trying to dial a new telephone number and someone starts talking to you about another topic, the new phone number may not register in your short-term memory, and you "forget" the number. Information needs to be held in short-term memory for a few seconds before it can be filed permanently into long-term memory. Distractions can also interfere with your attaching memory cues to the information, creating problems with your retrieving the information from long-term memory.

Uncorrected mechanical blocks can lead to more serious memory problems and a great deal of stress. Some memory aids can help lessen the impact of mechanical blocks.

- Get eyes and ears checked regularly.
- Keep glasses clean and hearing aids working.
- Remove distractions.
- Use all senses, and focus attention on information.
- Ask questions to improve understanding.
- Get rid of unnecessary information.
- Keep learning new things to keep the brain active.
- Remember new information by grouping similar things together.
- Make lists; post reminders on the refrigerator.
- Put important objects (keys, eyeglasses, etc.) in permanent places.
- Get rewards for remembering.

PHYSICAL BLOCKS

To function well, the brain needs to take in oxygen and get rid of wastes or toxins. The heart, lungs, liver, and kidneys work to carry out these vital functions. Because older adults have limited "reserves" for adapting to changes, these organs do not work as well under stress or when illness occurs. The decreased excretion or removal of toxins from the body makes older adults more sensitive to medications and their side effects including confusion. Older adults take an average of four to six medications, which are often prescribed by different physicians. All medications have side effects. Some medications should not be taken together because they have bad interactions. Your physician and nurse need to be aware of all medications the person is taking. Special precautions should be taken with all drugs, particularly tranquilizers, sedatives, sleeping pills, nicotine, and alcohol. These medications often cause confusion in older adults.

Most physical blocks to memory can be prevented or reversed by living healthier lifestyles. Various memory aids for physical blocks are important for you, the caregiver, as well as for the person receiving care.

- Quit smoking
- Drink six to eight glasses of water each day.
- Eat a low-fat diet with adequate vitamins and minerals.
- Exercise regularly, walking at least 15 minutes a day.
- Get on a regular sleeping schedule.
- Take medications as prescribed; minimize your use of sedatives, tranquilizers, and over-the-counter drugs.
- Keep a list of the names and dosages of your medications; take that list with you to the physician's office.
- Limit your alcohol intake.
- Get annual health screenings and check-ups.
- Report any sudden or persistent changes in memory or behavior that interfere with usual, daily functioning.

EMOTIONAL BLOCKS

Life changes and losses tend to multiply after age 65. Older adults usually are faced with adjusting to role changes, retirement, decreased financial resources, possible relocation, increased chronic health problems, and loss of family members and friends. These changes and losses make serious demands on the coping abilities of older adults. Feelings of depression, helplessness, anger, guilt, and fear are common. These emotional blocks play a big part in how and what we remember. There are some ways to get these emotional blocks under control and improve memory.

- Decide what helps you to relax and do that activity daily.
- Get rid of anger and guilt; some things need to be forgotten.
- Don't waste energy on the unimportant stresses.
- Keep a daily journal as a way to reflect on feelings and accomplishments.
- Set goals, and plan each day.

- Seek professional help if you continue to cope poorly with major stresses.
- Remember that memory is affected by mind, body, and spirit.
- Get rewards for coping and using problem solving.

FORGETFULNESS PROBLEMS

The person you are caring for may be experiencing more serious forgetfulness problems resulting from a combination of mechanical, physical, and emotional problems. If you are becoming concerned that the forgetfulness is becoming a threat to a person's ability to stay at home alone, a comprehensive physical examination is needed to rule out the presence of depression, delirium, or dementia. You can also help serious forgetfulness problems by making the environment more structured and safe with additional memory aids for specific problems. Involve the person receiving care in choices. For instance, if you are concerned about the person remembering to eat or to cook safely, there are several options. You can arrange "Meals on Wheels" to deliver one meal a day. If that service is not available, you might check on transportation to a senior center or church group for lunch. That choice would offer social benefits as well. You could also have a family member or friend bring in cooked food for the week.

Clocks, timers, and calendars can be used as reminders for daily activities. These types of additional memory aids may keep a person functioning independently. It is preferable to use these types of aids instead of your constantly reminding a person to do things. Depending on how serious the forgetfulness is, you may also need to check on the dependent person with calls or have a homemaker service.

The general guideline is to be as creative as you can in trying to find ways to help maintain the highest level of independence, sense of control, and dignity. If you continue to be worried about the safety of a person, you should seek a health professional's evaluation of the situation. The problem may be one of *confusion* rather than the forgetfulness problem of aging.

RECOGNIZING AND MANAGING THE THREE *D*s: DEPRESSION, DELIRIUM, AND DEMENTIA

DEPRESSION

Fortunately, we are hearing more about depression these days. It is coming out of the closet. For too long depression has been looked at as a "weakness" rather than a health problem that can be treated. In older adults the signs of depression can easily be missed. Depression can mimic the chronic confusion of dementia or the confusion caused by some medications and chronic illnesses.

The caregiver and the care receiver are both at risk for depression. Depression is more than the sadness or grief everyone experiences when they receive bad news. That type of sadness is normal. Review the following chart to see if you or the person you are caring for might be suffering from a clinical depression. If four or more of the following symptoms continue for more than two weeks, you need to call your physician:

- Feelings of emptiness, ongoing sadness, and anxiety.
- Lack of energy, tiredness, and fatigue.
- Loss of interest or pleasure in usual activities including sex.
- Sleep problems, either insomnia or excessive sleepiness.
- Eating problems, weight gain, or weight loss.
- Feeling worthless or guilty.
- Difficulty concentrating, remembering, or making decisions.
- Aches and pains that will not go away.
- Feeling restless or irritable.
- Frequent crying.
- Thoughts of death or suicide; suicide attempt.

Do not ignore these warning signs. If you notice them, get help. It is easy to think that problems with attention and memory are just signs of aging or signs of Alzheimer's disease, when they are actually a response to depression. Remember that depression is treatable in most cases. Antidepressant medications have become more and more effective with fewer side effects. These drugs are especially helpful when they are combined with short-term counseling. Clinical depression is an illness that will not go away by itself. It requires professional treatment, just as any other serious health problem does. If cost is a problem, community mental health centers can help. Call your physician or nurse to set up an evaluation and referral for treatment.

In addition to professional treatment, there are things you can do to help prevent depression. Plan for at least 30 minutes of daily exercise. Exercise will help your appetite, sleep, and general sense of well-being. Relaxation, positive self-talk, and laughter also need to be included in the daily routine. The information a few pages back about aids to emotional blocks should be helpful, too.

DELIRIUM

Delirium differs from depression and dementia in that it is an acute or sudden confusion. It can be life threatening. If you notice a sudden change in mental alertness and increased confusion, there is probably some newly developed physical problem. It could be an infection, even though an older adult may not have a fever. A lack of oxygen resulting from an acute cardiac or circulatory problem can also cause delirium. Many other things can upset the delicate balance within the body. Poor nutrition, insufficient fluid intake, imbalance of body chemicals, or side effects from medications are frequently involved. If the person receiving care has dementia already, adding delirium to it will increase the confusion and make caregiving more difficult.

People with dementia are at high risk for delirium. As a caregiver you need to be observant and suspicious of delirium whenever you see *sudden* changes in mental status and behavior. Some specific symptoms of delirium are fluctuations from drowsiness to restlessness, decreased alertness and more confusion, changes in sleep patterns, and mood changes. Notify the physician or nurse if you observe these sudden changes. The cause of delirium needs to be identified and treated quickly before permanent brain damage occurs.

The family caregiver knows the person receiving care much better than the physician or nurse does. Other caregivers need to work closely with family caregivers. Observations of changes in behavior should be communicated to health professionals. Chapter 2 contains information about ways to communicate effectively with health professionals. You need to be an advocate and make certain that the signs of delirium are fully evaluated. Delirium should not be dismissed as dementia. If the person receiving care is diagnosed as having delirium, important goals are to treat the cause of the delirium, restore the person's highest level of health, and maintain a safe environment. Hospitalization may be needed.

You can be an advocate for the person receiving care in the hospital setting. The hospital can be a frightening place for anyone, but especially so if a person has delirium and possibly dementia as well. The environment needs to be made as safe and least stressful as possible. Noise levels need to be controlled. The atmosphere needs to be calm and unrushed. Consistent staff should be assigned to care for the person. You can bring in some familiar objects to make the person feel securer. Help staff to know the patient as a person. Tell them about preferences and usual routines. You may be able to prevent agitation and the need for restraints. Physical restraints should be avoided and used as only a last resort. Research has shown that restraints have negative effects. They tend to increase confusion, agitation, and injury from falls.

DEMENTIA

Dementia is a progressive, debilitating, chronic confusion that slowly robs a person of memory and thinking abilities. Although about 3% of people younger than 65 years of age have problems with dementia, 18% of people between 75 to 84 years of age and 47% older than age 85 have some form of dementia. Most dementias are of the Alzheimer's type. Impaired circulation to the brain from small strokes (multiinfarct dementia) is a second major cause of dementia.

Alzheimer's disease progresses gradually from 1 to 10 years, with an average of 10 years, from the time of diagnosis until death. The cause of Alzheimer's disease is unknown. Although several drug studies are occurring, no medication currently exists that can stop the progression or reverse the deterioration of brain cells. You can check with the physician about any current investigational drug studies.

The course of this disease tends to progress through three stages.

First Stage

In the first stage, which lasts from 2 to 4 years, the symptoms may be so vague that no one is quite sure what is happening. The afflicted person tries hard to cover up the memory problems, but appears less energetic and has less drive or sparkle. It is not uncommon for depression to occur at this time because of the person's awareness of memory changes. Increased forgetfulness, loss of words, difficulty reading and learning, and angry outbursts become commoner as this stage progresses.

If the person you are caring for is in this stage of dementia, you will notice problems in his or her ability to carry out *instrumental activities of daily living,* such as cooking, driving, handling finances, taking medications, and so on. Safety becomes a serious concern. You may need to ask your physician for a referral to have a nurse visit the home to evaluate functional abilities and home safety. The Alzheimer's Association (see appendix) has extensive information about ways to handle specific situations. You might want to check with your local chapter for more information about support groups. The general guideline is to involve the care recipient in decisions to the extent possible, as you strive to create a safe environment and maintain the person's dignity and highest level of functioning.

Second Stage

During the second stage there is a definite memory loss, difficulty making decisions, and language problems. If you are caring for a person in this stage, you will need to supervise or assist him or her with the instrumental activities of daily living as well as basic activities, such as bathing, dressing, toileting, and so on. A person in this stage may become suspicious and agitated. Wandering behavior and other problem behaviors become more common. Ways to manage these behaviors will be discussed later in this chapter.

Last Stage

In the final stage of Alzheimer's disease or dementia, the affected person becomes highly disabled. This stage is characterized by disorientation to person, place, and time. There are also further changes in behavior. The affected person loses control of basic functions. Incontinence (loss of control of urine and bowel movements), mobility problems, eating problems, and communication problems increase. (Other chapters in this book deal with ways to manage those problems). As a caregiver of a person in this stage, you will have much difficulty accepting the loss of a relationship. It is also painful to discover the person no longer recognizes you. General deterioration progresses, with death often resulting from infections.

Most people with dementia are cared for at home by a family caregiver. The caregiving responsibilities are most difficult and often create physical, emotional, and financial burdens. In addition to the routine caregiving tasks of helping a dependent person with basic daily activities, behavior problems also occur as the dementia progresses. Caregiver depression and physical strain often result as the caregiving demands and the difficult behavioral changes increase. If you are caring for a person with dementia, seek out the support and help of others. You will have much difficulty if you attempt to care for the person alone. Read the information in Chapter 2 carefully about available community resources and making the nursing home decision. You need to care for yourself if you want to care for another person effectively.

MANAGING BEHAVIOR PROBLEMS

In this section, I discuss how to manage some of the commonest behavior problems that occur as the dementia progresses. These behaviors might also be seen with depression, delirium, or a combination of the three Ds. Managing the behavior problems can take a lot of your physical and emotional energy. It is important to remember that the behaviors are related to the brain changes. Internal or external stresses can cause the problem behaviors to come to the surface. The person has no control over these behaviors.

PREVENTION

Observe the person you are caring for closely for the warning signs of behavior problems and try to identify the causes. A good place to start is to consider internal stresses, which might bring about behavior problems. Be aware that persons with dementia are frail and more likely to become delirious from things like influenza and other respiratory and urinary infections. Their bones are more brittler and they have poor mobility skills. These conditions place them at risk for falls and fractures, which also increase delirium risks. Simple preventive measures can be taken to decrease the chances of health problems that can cause delirium and behavior problems. Some health prevention measures are getting annual flu shots; taking calcium or estrogen replacement; having regular eye and hearing examinations; maintaining good nutrition; setting up routines for exercise, toileting, and sleep; and controlling pain.

You will be able to prevent problems and identify better strategies for managing the behavior problems if you focus on the underlying cause of the problem. Also consider what the person is feeling at the time of the disruptive behavior. Do not get discouraged; disruptive behaviors are usually short-lived. Get help if you need it.

WANDERING BEHAVIOR

A common behavior problem, particularly during the middle stage of dementia, is wandering. Wandering can be aimless walking or walking to find someone, such as a parent who died several years ago. The confused person who wanders away from home or from a health care facility can be seriously injured. Safety is your primary concern. You may need to use an alarm or a lock on the door. Research has shown that putting a full-length mirror on the door keeps wandering persons away from the door. They do not recognize themselves in the mirror. They think another person is standing there. Also, covering up the door knobs with flowers or some other object disguises the door.

You can think of ways to make it more difficult to wander without using restraints. For example, you can use a recliner chair. You can also stretch out on the sofa with the person you are caring for sitting at one end. If you put your head in that person's lap, you'll create a warm connection, and you'll know when he or she gets up. A favorite television program or music may provide a distraction. Remember that the wandering behavior may be serving a purpose or meeting a need. The wandering often reduces anxiety and tension. Thus, your goal might be to reduce the wandering behavior but also to provide a safe area for wandering. Here are some things you can do for wandering behavior:

- Give the confused person a Med-Alert bracelet; register with the police the name and descriptive information about the person.
- Safety-proof the home; use alarms and locks on doors as needed.
- Put up simple signs, showing the person where to go and where not to go.
- Assist with toileting needs on a routine schedule.
- Use a recliner chair to make getting up to wander more difficult.
- Provide distractions (television, music, and pets) to keep attention off wandering.
- Provide regular exercise and a safe area for walking.
- Put a mirror on the door, or cover up the door knob to keep person from leaving the room.
- Surround the person with familiar things.
- Use a night light.
- Avoid changes in the environment.
- Approach quietly and calmly.
- Use sedatives and physical restraints as a last resort.

AGITATION

Agitation is a common problem and needs to be addressed quickly before it becomes aggressive behavior. Agitation can appear in the form of restlessness, wandering, disturbed sleep, or aggression. The underlying cause might be a physiological problem, such as an infection, cardiac problem, drug reaction, pain, constipation, and so on. It might also be brought on by a stressful event, such as relocation or a perception of harm. Loud noises or a rushed environment can also cause the person with confusion to become agitated. Agitation is made worse by using restraints. Again, restraints should be used as only a last resort and for only emergency situations. Problems with wandering, confusion, and agitation commonly get worse in the evening; this worsening is referred to as "sundowning." It is not known why sundowning occurs. It may be due to being tired and having less energy to cope with any changes. You will want to decrease activities and keep the environment quiet in the evening.

Here are some strategies you can use to prevent or reduce agitation.

- Remove the upsetting factors.
- Keep noise level down.
- Keep calm; do not shout.
- Keep things as simple as possible.
- Consider using soft music.
- Schedule 30-minute quiet periods in midmornings and afternoon; use an afghan as a sign for rest time.
- Give positive reinforcement for nonaggressive behavior.
- Get help if agitation changes to hostility.

The person receiving your care may also have problems with delusions or hallucinations, that is, seeing or hearing things that are not actually there. Do not try to contradict or correct. You will only increase distrust and agitation. Distraction would be a more useful strategy.

A WORD OF CAUTION ABOUT ELDER ABUSE

It takes a great deal of patience and energy to care for a person with chronic confusion, especially if agitation or combativeness is occurring. Give yourself permission to lose patience or get angry once in a while. But if you begin finding yourself yelling at the person receiving your care, ignoring basic needs, or striking out in anger, *get help immediately*.

Call a supportive friend or family member. Try to get some respite time. Talk with your physician or nurse. The Alzheimer's Association also can direct you to getting some help. Remember that loving, caring persons can become abusive or neglectful of a confused person. Keep that from happening. Seek reinforcement.

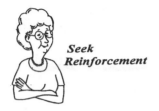

Seek Reinforcement

It is critical that you work closely with the physician, nurse, and other caregivers. You can provide valuable information, which will help in identifying the needed health care.

With the information in this chapter about confusion, you can use problem-solving skills in giving care. You have gained information about the differences in the mild forgetfulness of normal aging and the memory loss and confusion in the three *D*s: depression, delirium, and dementia. You have learned that a person can become affected by all three *D*s at the same time. A frail elderly person with chronic confusion or dementia is at high risk for the three *D*s. It is important to identify the differences and treat the causes of the problem. It may not always be possible to reverse the cause, but there are many strategies that can be used to improve comfort, functioning, and quality of life.

Caring for a person who is confused takes its toll on the caregiver. Learn about all the resources available in your community. Take all the help you can get from family and friends. Take time out for yourself, the caregiver. Draw on the resources of the Alzheimer's Association. Read other books about Alzheimer's disease, especially ones that give you more insight into the feelings of the affected person. *The Loss of Self* by Donna Cohen and Carl Eisdorfer is one such book you might want to read.

5

Comfort and Pain Control

Ann Schmidt Luggen

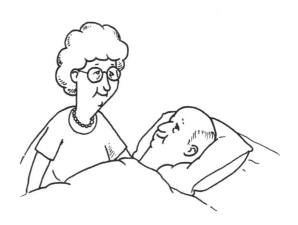

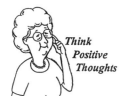

Think Positive Thoughts

Pain is not a normal consequence of aging, but it accompanies many of the chronic health problems that occur frequently as we age. You, as a caregiver of someone with a great deal of pain, may struggle with how to help. Actually, there are many things that you can do to make the person you are caring for more comfortable as well as reduce the pain.

Older adults receiving care do not need to suffer needlessly. In this chapter, I discuss some of the common causes of pain and how to reduce the pain right in your own home. I will also show you how to keep a written record of the pain, so that you can describe it better when you talk to the physician or nurse about medications and other treatments that can help. I am going to help you learn about pain and how you can help the person receiving care to deal with pain. Take a deep breath, and get comfortable before you read this information.

PAIN IN OLDER ADULTS

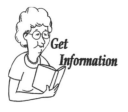 *Get Information*

Although researchers have studied pain a great deal in the past 20 years, relatively little has been studied about pain in older adults. Some people think that because elderly people lose some of their sensory abilities (e.g., seeing, smelling, and tasting), they lose their pain sensations as well. Also, because elderly people have painful chronic illnesses, such as arthritis, many people believe that they adjust easily to the pain. There is no evidence that this is so. In fact, although elderly people seem to perceive pain *differently* from the way younger adults do, several research studies have found that older adults are suffering needlessly and living with considerable pain on a daily basis.

Physicians and nurses may also have mistaken ideas about pain in older people, and they may not prescribe enough pain medications. They may also be concerned about how the pain medicine will affect the older person who may already be taking several medications. The result is that older adults often endure pain when they do not need to suffer. When pain medicine is needed, older adults should be encouraged to take the proper dosage of that medicine.

TYPES OF PAIN

There are two major kinds of pain: acute and chronic pain. Acute pain is usually caused by an injury or surgery. This pain is sharp and severe, but ceases in a few days or weeks. It is usually treated with strong-acting analgesics or drugs that take away pain. Chronic pain is the pain you have with such problems as arthritis. It begins gradually and lasts a long time, perhaps forever. Chronic pain responds well to a combination of medications and treatment that help to reduce pain and inflammation, and the depression or stress that chronic pain may cause. Both kinds of pain can exist at the same time.

RESPONSES TO PAIN

People respond to pain in different ways. Pain can change a person's behavior. Sometimes, people who are warm, gentle, and outgoing may become irritable and withdrawn.

Another very common response to pain, especially long-lasting pain, is depression. People who are depressed feel less interested in the things they used to enjoy. They look sad. They may have a change in appetite, either increased or decreased. They may not sleep well or may moan or be very restless. When depression becomes severe, people feel worthless and may think about death or suicide. At this point, they are feeling almost no control over the pain. These people need professional help right away. People with pain need to feel they have some control over the pain. There are prescribed medications that help both depression and chronic pain. You need to ask the physician or nurse about these medications.

Pain can also interfere with a person's ability to get around as they use to. They may not be able to do the everyday things, such as brushing teeth or buttoning buttons. Being dependent is very frustrating and adds to the irritability that may already be present from the pain, making the whole situation worse. You may need to convince the person you are caring for to let you help. You need to make them feel that you want to help and that you enjoy being able to help. Giving up one's independence is not an easy thing to do.

WAYS TO KEEP DEPENDENT OLDER
ADULTS COMFORTABLE

One of the best ways to keep a person comfortable is *to be there*. I know that can be very difficult to do, especially if he or she is irritable or moaning. People who have chronic pain, even though they isolate themselves, often fear being abandoned. Just having you there is a comfort.

Some people with chronic pain may need to have pain medication around the clock, for example, every 4 hours during the day *and* night hours. That means that you don't wait until they cry out or moan. Pain is much easier to prevent than it is to stop it after it starts.

You can ask the physician about giving pain medications, such as Tylenol, every 4 hours so the pain never gets very bad. This schedule can be followed along with other stronger pain medications. You can often reduce the number of stronger pain medications, if you keep the pain lessened with drugs such as acetaminophen (Tylenol), aspirin, or ibuprofen (Motrin or Advil). Remember that older adults are more sensitive to medications, so make sure you discuss any new medications you give with the physician or nurse.

It is important to have the pain medication at its peak *before* you move or bathe the person. "At its peak" means the time when the medication is the strongest and most effective. Most medications that you give by mouth take 20 minutes or so to take effect. Even if you are giving around-the-clock pain medications, at the end of the 4 hours, the pain medication is less effective. You want to schedule the turning, the bath, or getting up to the chair, for a time when the medication is at its peak. Usually, the peak time is 1 or 2 hours after giving the pain medication. You will know when the peak time is because the person will be most comfortable at the time. Also, if you have a second, stronger medication you can give, then give that stronger medication about 1 hour or so before moving the person for daily activities.

One of the ways to add comfort is to keep the person receiving care clean and dry. Some people perspire a lot, especially during painful episodes. Damp clothing and sheets can be very uncomfortable and irritating to the skin. Many older adults have skin that is dry and flaky, and it may be itchy. Itchiness, when added to pain, makes the pain worse. Rubbing a soothing lotion on the skin will help if it is dry and itchy. Actually, any unpleasant or uncomfortable situation makes pain worse. You can bathe the older adult in bed, if getting up is too painful.

If the person is able to get up and get into a tub, a warm bath is one of the best things for mild to moderate pain. A warm bath is soothing and relaxing, and can make stiff joints more mobile, less painful. Just as warm water can be very helpful in reducing pain for some people, for others, cool or cold can reduce pain. A cold bath is not a good idea, but cool compresses on a joint, such as the knee, elbow, or wrist, may reduce pain considerably. A joint that is warm and red and swollen will often feel much better with this kind of comfort measure.

Another way to keep a person comfortable is to keep the environment pleasant. Avoid loud, irritating noises. Play soothing music to distract attention from the pain. If the person enjoys television, radio programs, or the newspaper, have them available in the room.

Other ideas to add comfort include having a glass of fresh water close at hand, keeping the room temperature comfortable, and having a blanket handy. Ask the person what he or she needs to be comfortable.

RECOGNIZING WHEN PAIN MEDICATIONS ARE NEEDED

Some people are uncomfortable about taking pain medications. They have fears about becomes addicted. The fact is, when people have painful conditions, it is extremely rare for anyone to become addicted. Less than half of 1% of people who take prescribed narcotics become addicted. People who are in pain need pain relief. For certain cancers that may be very painful and for acute pain after surgery, narcotics are often preferred to nonnarcotic drugs. The narcotic drug may actually have fewer side effects than the other pain medications, and it will bring relief that other medications cannot provide.

How do you know if a person needs pain medication? Not everyone will tell you that they are in pain. Not everyone moans or cries with pain. Some people, and especially older adults, have learned to hold in their pain. They have been told to be brave. You probably know the person you are caring for well enough to know if he or she is this kind of person. The best way is to find out if a person is having pain is to ask, "Are you comfortable?" Many older adults think of pain as "discomfort" rather than as "pain."

Some people may go to sleep, and you think that because they are sleeping, they must not have pain. This is not necessarily the case.

Just as some people isolate themselves because of pain, some people try to escape from the pain by sleeping. It is not usually a restful, deep sleep, and they do not feel fresh and rested afterward. It is better to give the pain medication if you notice that the sleep is light or restless.

As I mentioned, a change in behavior may be a sign a person is having pain. If a person withdraws or stops doing the things he or she previously enjoyed, you can be fairly certain that pain is present.

The best thing you can do to learn whether the pain is being helped by the pain medications or other treatments is to ask the person, "How is your pain (or discomfort)?" Ask the person to rate how strong the pain is on a scale of 0 to 10, with 0 meaning no pain at all and 10 meaning the worst pain you can ever imagine. You can ask this question before giving the pain medication, and you can ask again before giving the next dose. If the pain medication is not working at the present dose, you may want to call the physician about increasing the dose or giving it a little sooner than it has been prescribed.

If the pain on the scale (0–10) is a 5 or 6, it is too much pain (see Figure 5.1). It is moderate pain and means the pain medication is not working very well.

Other pain treatments, such as massage, and heat or cold treatments, do not help when the pain is at this level. If the pain is 3 or less, it is mild pain, and the other techniques mentioned previously will work.

If the pain is getting worse before the next dose is due, ask the physician about changing the schedule or the dose. The physician may also change the medication or combine the narcotic with another pain reliever.

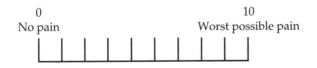

FIGURE 5.1 Pain scale.

SIDE EFFECTS FROM MEDICATIONS

Over-the-counter pain medications or the ones you buy without a prescription are used for mild to low-moderate pain. Examples are aspirin, ibuprofen, and acetaminophen. These drugs also have side effects or effects other than helping the pain. Aspirin and ibuprofen can cause stomach upset and need to be taken with food. They can also cause bleeding, which can become serious. If you see some blood oozing from a scratch for a long time or if you see blood in the bowel movement, you need to call the physician or nurse to find out what they want you to do. If you give large doses of aspirin (8–12 aspirins or more a day), ringing in the ears can occur. This unpleasant side effect should go away when you decrease or stop the aspirin.

Your doctor many prescribe narcotic drugs simply because these are very effective in relieving pain. These medications also have side effects, so you will need to watch for them so they do not cause problems.

Drowsiness is a very common side effect of narcotics. This side effect can help promote sleep, but it can also increase the risk of falling. Usually, the drowsiness occurs just when the narcotic treatment is started and goes away in a few days.

Constipation is another very common side effect of narcotic drugs. The best thing to do is to increase fluids unless fluids are restricted for some other reason. Also, give more foods with fiber. The doctor may order a stool softener to use with narcotic medications. Nausea and even vomiting may occur with these pain medications. Nausea and vomiting make a person in pain even more miserable. Sometimes the nausea and vomiting are caused by an illness, but it can also be caused by the medications. Nausea with narcotics usually lasts about 3 days. During that time, the doctor can give something for nausea.

Slow, shallow breathing can occur with narcotic medications. If you think this is happening, the person is probably on too high a dose or is taking the drug too often. Medications stay in the body a longer time in older people. They can build up in the body. You may need to delay the next dose of the drug or skip it, as long as the pain is under control. Check with the physician or nurse about changing the dose or schedule for the medication.

TABLE 5.1 Pain Medication Record

Date/ time	Medication	Dose or amount	Amount of pain (0–10) scale	Side effects

If you are using an antidepressant medication, some side effects to watch for are dry mouth, difficulty with urination, blurry vision, or dizziness. You can give frequent sips of water for the dry mouth. A lip balm may be comforting, too.

Write down any side effects, and let the physician or nurse know about them. Table 5.1 is an example of a record you can use to keep track of pain medications and how they are working.

ALTERNATIVE PAIN-RELIEVING TREATMENTS

HEAT TREATMENTS

Heat promotes healing. It is often used for acute pain, but many people with rheumatoid arthritis use warm baths to get going in the morning. It seems to relax their stiff, painful joints. Some people cannot start the day without this important treatment. If the person you are caring for has a sprain or a muscle spasm, applying moist heat for 15 to 20 minutes at a time can be very beneficial in relieving pain. Be sure to check the temperature of the water or heating pad, particularly with older persons, who might not feel hot temperatures as well.

COLD TREATMENTS

Cold is numbing. You will see that it also reduces the redness and swelling to the applied area. Cold treatments are especially useful treatments right after an injury such as a fall or a sprain. Apply the cold for about 15 to 20 minutes each time you use it. If you use ice cubes, put them in a plastic bag, sealed tightly, and wrap the bag in a towel or cloth. Ice can injure the skin without this protection. For some people, cold treatments are very unpleasant, and you won't want to use cold even if you know it will help. Some of the feelings people have with cold treatments are a feeling of cold, then a feeling of burning, then aching, and then numbness. These feelings with cold treatments are normal. You may recall some of these feelings when you have been outside in cold weather, and your hand or foot becomes numb.

RELAXATION

Relaxation can serve as a pain-relief treatment and a comfort measure for the person receiving care, as well as for you. Pain causes people to become tense. Tense muscles become painful. In this way, tenseness increases the pain. Relaxation techniques are helpful for both acute and chronic pain, especially if the pain is mild to low-moderate pain (ranging between 2 and 4 on a 0–10 scale). Some of the other treatments I've already discussed, including medications, will help get the pain under control so that relaxation can be most beneficial.

Breathing exercises are one way to relax. Practice the following two exercises before you teach them to the person receiving your care, so that you know how they work:

Exercise 1

Drop your jaw (as if you were going to yawn).

- Breathe slowly and evenly.
- Try to stop thinking, and just try to maintain this state of relaxed jaw and slow, even breathing.

Exercise 2

- Take a deep breath slowly.
- Blow out the air slowly, thinking that all anxiety and tension are flowing out with the breath.
- Repeat several times until you feel less tension and anxiety.

Imagery is another technique to use after you have gotten relaxed with the breathing techniques. Imagery seems to give the person with pain a sense of control. It also reduces pain by reducing anxiety and tension and takes the person's mind away from the pain. Imagery is done several ways. My favorite is to recall a time and a place that brings back pleasant, happy memories. For example, you might picture yourself at the beach. You can recall the soft warm sands beneath your bare feet. You can feel the gentle warm winds from the ocean and the rolling waves that are endlessly lapping at the beach. You can even hear the waves lapping at the shore and smell the salty air. In this imagery practice, you can see, hear, smell, and feel that special place. You can relive the feelings and experiences deep within yourself and feel relaxed and happier.

DISTRACTIONS

Distractions also work very well for mild to medium pain. They do not work for severe pain, which needs to be treated with medication.

Television is one of the best distractions for mild pain. It occupies the mind's thoughts so that one does not think about pain. Usually during a commercial, the pain will be perceived again. As with music, you must find a program that the person enjoys. You may find with television or music that the volume of the program may be varied, depending on how severe the pain is at the time. Low volume can be used with very mild pain and louder volume with moderate pain.

Reading can help for mild pain. The reading material content should be the kind of material the person likes to read. You can read to the pain sufferer, or for very mild pain, the person may want to read by himself or herself. It is a good distraction, especially if it is a good story.

Sleep is a distractor of pain, even severer pain. Sleep may come easily when a person is exhausted from pain. The sleep takes people away from the pain, although the pain is still there. A quiet, comfortable setting promotes sleep.

Activity keeps you distracted from pain. It doesn't really matter what the activity is—taking a bath, drawing, writing, visiting with a friend, talking to children, or petting a kitten. See if you can come up with a list of distraction activities.

OTHER PAIN-RELIEF MEASURES

There are many other ways to help a person find relief from pain. These alternatives will require outside help, and you can ask your nurse or physician about these options. One example is *hypnosis*. Hypnosis can work very well, even for severer pain. Some people can learn to hypnotize themselves, but it will have to be taught by an expert. Some people can by hypnotized by another person for pain relief.

Another method of pain relief is *acupuncture*. This treatment for pain has been used for thousand of years and can be very successful. It requires a specialist to insert and manipulate tiny needles, which do not hurt. There is no feeling at all from the tiny needles. This pain management is being done increasingly, and so it would not be too difficult to find someone to do this.

A similar method is called *acupressure*. It is very much like acupuncture except without the needles. In the same places where needles would be inserted, the health professional (doctor, nurse, or other professional person) will apply firm, but gentle, pressure for several minutes until the pain is gone.

Another method of pain relief is *TENS unit*. This small device transmits electrical nerve stimulation (TENS is an acronym for *transcutaneous electric nerve stimulation*). The TENS unit stimulation competes with the pain stimulation and blocks the pain feelings. These devices can be very useful in relieving pain. They are available through your physician and can be rented. It is something you could try if other methods are not working very well.

There are people available in most towns who will come to your home to do *massage therapy*. It is a treatment that removes the tension that accompanies pain. It relaxes many people enough so that they sleep very well. It is especially useful for back pain and for pain in the jaw joint, just under the ear. If a person is unable to get exercise, massage is a useful way to stimulate the muscles and tissues.

One last pain-relief measure that I will mention you can do yourself. It is called *range-of-motion exercises,* and it is very helpful for people who are not getting any exercise because of the pain and their limited ability to get around. You know that if you sit for a long time or even when you get up in the morning, you are likely to become stiff, and your joints are painful. If the person receiving care cannot get up and around, this is even more stiffening and painful. You can gently move the joints of the fingers of his hand, rotating them back and forth. Move the joints within the range that they are able to move without causing pain. Move the joints of the hands, arms, legs, and feet. One example of what you can do just for the hand is making a fist with the hand. Then open the fist fully and hold it. Repeat. Then take each finger starting with the thumb, and move it every way that it can be moved: forward, sideways, or bent at the joint. Move each finger separately in this fashion. This is range of motion. It is helpful to do these 2-3 times every day.

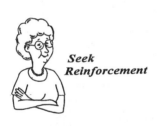

Seek Reinforcement

Let's review some of the key points we have discussed. The experience of pain in older adults is not well understood by health professionals. Many people have the misconception that it is a normal part of aging. Pain is treated with less attention in older adults, and, as a consequence, there is much needless suffering. In fact, there is much that can be done to alleviate pain and promote comfort. Although there are many things you can do alone as a caregiver, it is better to work together on a plan with the physician or nurse.

As a caregiver, you also might need to use the comfort and relaxation measures for yourself. They can help you relax, feel more in control of the situation, and have more energy. And, most of all, you can feel that you are doing something important to help and support another person because you are.

Just remember, you can try many things to control pain and make someone more comfortable. You are not alone. There are many resources you can call on. Work with your physician and nurse to discover what works best for the care recipient and, perhaps, for you. In the appendix of this book is a list of several organizations that will provide you with information about resources in your community.

6

Promoting Mobility and Preventing Falls

Alicia Curtin

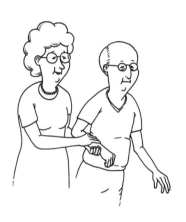

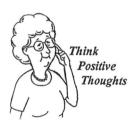

Think Positive Thoughts

Many people think we need to slow down and take it easy as we get older. They also believe that physical decline is inevitably associated with aging. However, for many of us this is not true. Physical decline can sometimes be caused by disuse and inactivity rather than by advancing age. Also, many mobility problems associated with chronic diseases or aging can be delayed or slowed down by doing regular exercise. Actually, regular exercise can have many beneficial effects. It can improve mood, reduce stress and tension, help with sleeping better at night, control weight, improve strength and mobility, reduce blood pressure, and increase the circulation to legs and feet. Exercise is especially important for the dependent older adult who may be at risk for immobility.

So, take a deep breath now, inhale slowly, and exhale slowly, as we look at how aging changes in the body can affect our mobility.

AGING CHANGES AND CHRONIC DISEASES AFFECTING MOBILITY

As we grow older, our bodies go through many changes. These changes vary from person to person because of our different

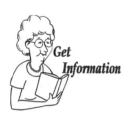
Get Information

lifestyles and the traits we have inherited from our ancestors. Few changes are caused solely by growing older. For example, some people have a family history of diabetes. This health condition may be inherited. Other health conditions are influenced by the way we have lived our lives. People can be at greater risk for cardiac disease because of their family history, but cardiac disease is also more common in people who are inactive, are overweight, smoke, and eat a high-fat diet. Thus, the development of chronic diseases, whether inherited or influenced by our lifestyle habits, will have an affect on our bodies as we grow older.

Most age-related changes are due to inactivity and deconditioning. Knowing about these changes will allow us to take action to decrease their influences on our daily activities.

- Decrease in muscle strength and flexibility.
- Decrease in endurance.
- Decrease in height and bone mass.
- Stiffening of joints.
- Decrease in lung expansion.
- Decrease in balance.

- Decrease in vision and hearing.
- Mild increase in blood pressure.

Chronic diseases also affect our ability to move freely. Osteo-arthritis may cause pain and stiffness in joints, making it difficult to walk, get up from a chair or bed, and perform certain activities we enjoy. Osteoporosis causes bones to become brittle and break easily. Heart and lung diseases may limit our ability to walk even short distances or perform such activities as bathing and dressing. Muscle weakness from a stroke may make it more difficult to walk without some type of assistance. Diabetes may cause numbness and tingling in the hands and feet, making it more difficult to walk. Dementia and other diseases that cause memory problems may lead to mobility problems because of inability following directions or forgetting how to walk. Poor eyesight, hearing, and sense of touch may affect a person's balance and ability to walk safely without falling.

Regardless of these age-related changes and changes resulting from chronic disease, a regular routine of exercise or body movement can keep us flexible and strong and slow down the aging process.

PROPER POSITIONING AND TRANSFERRING

Taking care of someone at home, especially someone having problems with moving around independently, can be very frustrating. Remember, you are not alone. There are many physically disabled people living at home. Some people learn how to transfer and walk with help from family members or friends or by using an assistive device. An assistive device is any type of equipment that helps someone to move around more independently. Examples are a wheelchair, walker, or cane. Other assistive devices may help to lift or move someone who may have complete inability to move on their own.

Before learning more about the devices that can help you, it is important to learn about the people who can help you. Your doctor and nurse can be valuable resources for this information. Your doctor or nurse can refer you to a physical therapist. The physical therapist can assess the disabled person's ability to transfer and walk safely. They can also assess the person's need for an assistive device and will teach the person how to use such a device. If the person you are caring for needs physical assistance, the physical therapist will teach you how to help without straining your back.

Assistive devices can make your job of moving or lifting someone a lot easier. For example, a draw sheet can be used to help move someone in bed. A draw sheet is a heavy cotton sheet that is placed under the person in bed. By grabbing hold of the draw sheet at the level of the person's shoulder and hip, you can move the disabled person from side to side or up toward the head of the bed.

A mechanical lift can also be used to transfer a person who is unable to move at all. A sturdy sling is placed under the disabled person in bed. Then, with a pumping action, the mechanical lift can be made to raise the person from the bed, position the person over a chair, and then guide the person into the chair. Although it sounds complicated, it is very easy and greatly reduces strain on your back. However, this equipment is very expensive. Some insurance companies may pay for such equipment if the transfer requires the assistance of two people and if without the use of a lift the person would be confined to bed.

Another device used to transfer an unsteady person is a transfer belt. The transfer belt fits around the disabled person's waist to give you a good handhold. The transfer belt is helpful when moving someone from the bed to a chair or when holding on to someone who is an unsteady walker. The physical therapist or nurse can teach you how to use each of these devices properly and safely.

Other assistive devices, as well as canes, walkers, and wheelchairs, can be ordered through medical supply companies. The physical therapist or nurse can also help you to order the proper equipment. Some equipment is covered by insurance, depending on the disabled person's medical needs.

The most important rule to learn when you are moving, lifting, or transferring someone is to use good body mechanics. Here are some key points to remember about body mechanics:

- Keep your feet apart for a wide base of support.
- Bend at the knees when lifting to have the large muscles in your legs do the work.

- Keep your back straight.
- Shift your weight from one leg to the other when lifting and moving.

There are three basic transfers that the physical therapist or nurse will teach you, depending on the disabled person's ability to move. These transfers are moving a person in bed, moving a person from the bed to a chair and back, and moving a person from a wheelchair or chair to the commode (portable toilet) or the toilet and back.

MOVING A PERSON IN BED

Moving a person in bed can be very easy if you know the right techniques. Always remember to use good body mechanics with any move. To pull a person up in bed, make sure the head of the bed is down. At the same time, you should grasp the draw sheet at the level of the person's shoulder and hip. Point your foot closest to the head of the bed, in the direction you are moving the person. Use your legs and body weight, by shifting your weight from one leg to the other. At the same time, ask the person in bed to bend their knees and push down with their feet on the count of three. On the count of three, lift and pull the person up in bed. If the disabled person is not able to help you, you may need two people or the mechanical lift to be successful.

To turn a person over in bed, you need to get as close as possible to the disabled person. Put the head of the bed down. Bend the person's leg that is farther away from you. Grasp the draw sheet on the other side at the level of the person's shoulder and hip, and turn the person toward you. Try to use the rest of your body more than your back.

MOVING A PERSON FROM BED

Moving a person from the bed to a chair often requires the disabled person's help. If the person is unable to help you, do not try to move him or her by yourself. Remember to never lift or move someone at the expense of your own back. Ask for help!

Always begin by explaining each move to the person. This will reassure the person and make the move smoother. The bed should be at its lowest height. Move the chair close to the bed. Turn the person on his or her side facing toward you in bed. Place your hand at the bottom of the disabled person's neck, resting your palm on the person's shoulder blade. Place your other hand under the person's knees. Swing the person's legs over the edge of the bed, helping the person to sit up. After you have the person sitting, ask them to scoot to the edge of the bed. The person's feet should be flat on the floor. Place the transfer belt around the person's waist. With your feet apart, grab hold of the transfer belt on each side. Ask the person to use his or her arms to push off the bed. On the count of three, lean back, shift your weight, lift, and pivot toward the chair. Have the person grab hold of the arms of the chair. Bend your knees, and lower the disabled person into the chair.

MOVING A PERSON FROM A WHEELCHAIR OR CHAIR TO A TOILET

When moving a person from a wheelchair or chair to the toilet, you will use the same technique as described earlier. Before beginning the move, make sure the wheelchair wheels are locked and cannot move. Have the person scoot to the edge of the chair. Make sure the disabled person's feet are flat on the floor. Grab the transfer belt in back. On the count of three, lean back, shift your weight, lift, and pivot in front of the toilet. Bend your knees, and lower the person down onto the toilet. When performing any transfers, remember to stand close to the person you are moving. This will prevent falls and reduce your risk for back injury.

TAKING CARE OF YOUR BACK

Not only is it important to learn the proper techniques for lifting and moving, but it is important to learn how to take care of your back. Self-care activities, such as back exercises and relaxation techniques, can help strengthen your back muscles and reduce stress and strain in your life. Take a few minutes each day to stretch your back. Lay flat on the floor, and bring your knees up to your chin.

Hold this position for 10 seconds, then release. Do this five times. This is an exercise that will help stretch your back muscles. Partial sit-ups will also help strengthen the muscles of your stomach and prevent back injury. Lie flat on the floor, bend your knees, arms stretched out in front of you, and lift your torso off the floor using your abdominal muscles. These types of exercises will warm up your body and prepare you for the activities of the day. Do these exercises two or three times a day to help you relax and clear your head.

Deep breathing is a technique that can also help you clear your head and focus on the job you need to do. Breathe in slowly and deeply, then exhale slowly and fully. Another relaxation technique is called visualization. Close your eyes and visualize a peaceful scene that will take your mind off your daily tasks and help you to relax. Do this visualization along with your deep breathing at least 5 to 10 minutes at the start of each day.

If you have back pain, do not perform any lifting or transfers. Rest your back. Apply ice to your back for 15 to 20 minutes, several times a day. This may help reduce the pain. Gentle back stretches can prevent stiffness and increase flexibility. If the pain persists or is severe, see your doctor.

EXERCISE

Exercise is important at any age! Many people believe that they need to slow down and take it easy as they age, but that is not the case. There are many benefits to exercising. Regular exercise can help strengthen your heart and lungs, reduce your blood pressure, reduce tension, and help you to sleep more restfully at night. Exercise can also protect against the problems associated with chronic diseases like diabetes, arthritis, osteoporosis, hypertension, and depression. It does not matter if a person has memory, mobility, or physical problems. Based on the persons' needs and skills, an exercise program can be designed for them. Exercise is one of the best things you can do for your health and the health of the person who you are caring for. Thus, the following information on exercise is not only to promote a regular exercise routine for the care recipient but also for you, the caregiver.

Sometimes it is difficult to start exercising, especially when you have not been active. Talk to your doctor before you or the person you are caring for begins any regular exercise program. Once you get started, try to stick to it. Set a special time during the day to make exercise a part of your daily routine.

Don't try to do too much at first. Go at your own speed, and slowly increase your level of activity. A goal should be about 30 minutes of exercise a day. However, you don't have to do that all at once. You can do 10 minutes of a certain activity three times a day, whether it's taking a 10 minute walk, vacuuming, or marching in place. Any type of routine exercise will help improve your health. Many exercises that improve flexibility and strength can be done during routine personal care like bathing and dressing. These exercises are important especially for the person you are caring for who is unsteady or is unable to move at all. These exercises will prevent contractures (tightening of the joints), pain, and muscle weakness.

The amount and type of exercise depends on your needs and the needs of the person for whom you are caring. There are two types of exercise: aerobic and low intensity. Aerobic exercise will strengthen your heart and lungs and improve overall fitness. Aerobic exercises include jogging, biking, walking briskly, and skiing. Low-intensity exercise will help control weight, prevent the loss of bone mass associated with osteoporosis, and improve muscle strength and flexibility. Low-intensity exercises will have little effect on strengthening the heart and lungs. Low-intensity exercises include walking, bowling, vacuuming, and gardening.

The components of an effective exercise program include stretching, strength training, and aerobics. Begin with stretching and strength training, and then add aerobics later. Aerobics are easier once you feel balanced and steady on your feet.

Stretching will improve flexibility and reduce the strain and injury of your muscles. Any type of exercise routine should begin with a 5- to 10-minute warm-up period of stretching and end with a 5- to 10-minute cool down. Stretching can help loosen the muscles in your neck, arms, legs, buttocks, back, calves, and thighs. These warm-up exercises will also prepare your body for the activities of the day.

Strength-training exercises will help strengthen muscles and bones. Strengthening exercises may include lifting weights or working out with weight machines or Theraband, a special type of elastic band. These types of exercises can improve your upper and lower body strength. Before beginning any strengthening program, talk with a physical therapist or exercise expert, who can show you the different strengthening that you should do. You do not have to buy any special equipment to begin your program. You can use household products, such as soup cans, milk jugs, or books that you can lift easily five times, bending at the elbow; rest a few minutes and repeat. You have completed two sets of repetitions. When you are able to do two sets easily, do three sets. Slowly increase the number of repetitions from 5 to 10 to 15. Once you are able to do three sets of 15 repetitions, slowly increase the amount of weight you are lifting.

You do not have to do strength training every day, nor do you have to use heavy weights to see the benefits. Generally, 30 minutes three times a week with light weights is sufficient. Be careful not to overdo it. You may injure your muscles if you exercise the same muscle groups two days in a row without a rest.

Stretching and strengthening exercises can be done in bed, in a chair, or even during your own personal care activities, like bathing and dressing. Also, encouraging disabled persons to comb their hair, tie shoes, and get dressed can help prevent muscle stiffness and joint tightness, called contractures. It is important to encourage the disabled person to do as much for themselves as they can.

Sometimes the person you are caring for won't be able to exercise, bathe, or dress because of physical or memory problems. There are still ways that you can help that person to exercise. If there is a memory problem, demonstrate a specific exercise first, then ask the person you are caring for to do the same. For example, raise your hands over your head and ask, "Can you do this?" If the person is unable to perform the specific movement, you can help. Using your hands, gently move the disabled person's arm, leg, or foot through its full range of motion. As you are doing the range-of-motion exercises, have the person breathe slowly and deeply and then exhale. Range-of-motion exercises will help to prevent contractures, joint and muscle pain, and muscle weakness for the person who is in bed or a wheelchair.

Improving the strength of a person confined to bed or a wheelchair can be difficult. However, your physical therapist or nurse can show you some strengthening exercises using Theraband, a type of elastic band. The elastic band can be tied to the foot of the bed and the disabled person can pull on it. These types of exercises will improve muscle strength and muscle tone.

Other types of strengthening exercises include low-intensity exercises like walking, gardening, bowling, and vacuuming. One of the safest and best low-intensity exercises is walking. Walking can be done anywhere, at anytime, and cost close to nothing. The only cost is to buy comfortable shoes with good support. Walking gives you and the person you are caring for the opportunity to get out of the house and get some fresh air. Walking improves muscle tone and reduces stress and tension.

If the weather is bad, you can walk or march in the house. Play some music and march to the rhythm of the music. Local malls, community centers, YMCAs, and YWCAs generally have some type of exercise or walking program that you can join. This is a great time to socialize and meet other people who may have the same physical problems with which you are dealing.

Aerobic exercises, such as biking, swimming, jogging, and walking briskly, is sometimes more difficult, but will strengthen the muscles of your heart and lungs. These types of activities will improve your endurance. Endurance is the ability to do an activity for longer periods without becoming tired. You may get some conditioning results from walking at normal speed, but it will take longer to reach this. By increasing your pace, increasing your distance, and increasing the frequency of walking, you can obtain the benefits of aerobic conditioning.

Remember, if you or the person you are caring for have any chest pain, shortness of breath, dizziness, or severe joint pain, *stop* the activity and check with your doctor.

The key to exercising regularly is to start slowly. Gradually increase the amount of exercise you do over time. Always breathe deeply throughout every type of exercise that you do. Remember to warm up for 5 to 10 minutes before any exercise program. Never stop an activity abruptly. End with 5 to 10 minutes of stretching exercises to cool down. Once these activities are part of your daily routine, you will see how easy it is to preserve flexibility and strength.

Several agencies offer free information on exercise. The National Institute on Aging offers free information on a variety of topics related to health and aging. A fitness book for older adults is obtainable through the American Association of Retired Persons' Health Promotion Service. Finally, contact your local library for books or videotapes about exercise and aging.

PROBLEMS OF IMMOBILITY

Many problems may occur if a person is immobile or inactive. Most of the physical decline associated with aging is due to inactivity, not the aging process. Persons at greatest risk for immobility-related health problems are those with memory or physical impairments resulting from chronic diseases.

For example, a person with dementia may be fearful of walking or even forget how to walk. A person with severe joint pain from arthritis may choose not to walk because of the pain. A person with muscle weakness resulting from a stroke may need assistance to perform daily activities. Whatever the reason, if a person has mobility problems, you as the caregiver need special assistance. Work with your doctor, nurse, and physical therapist. Together you can help the disabled person become more active and thereby prevent the problems caused by immobility.

Many medical problems are associated with inactivity and immobility. Pressure ulcers are skin sores that develop when a person sits or lies in the same position for too long. To prevent this problem, persons who are unable to move at all require repositioning every 2 hours. Repositioning takes the pressure off the involved area and allows the blood to circulate. Special care must be taken to assess the disabled person's skin daily for redness or breakdown. Proper nutrition and fluid intake are also very important for preventing pressure ulcers.

The immobile person is also at risk for infections. Pneumonia is more likely because the immobile person is not breathing deeply and expanding the lungs. Urinary tract infection is another common problem. A person using a bedpan may not empty their bladder completely, which may lead to an infection and leakage of urine (urinary incontinence).

Other common problems associated with immobility are muscle weakness and joint contractures. This overall deconditioning will make it difficult for the disabled person to regain the ability to dress, bathe, and transfer. If deconditioning sets in, the disabled person will become more dependent on the caregiver for these types of activities.

Still other common problems associated with immobility are constipation, depression, swelling of the legs, osteoporosis, weight loss or weight gain, decreased endurance, dizziness, and social isolation. These problems can be prevented by identifying the cause of immobility and helping the person to become more active. Even a small improvement in flexibility, strength, and endurance may have a great effect on a person's ability to perform basic activities of daily living. Disabled persons should be encouraged to do as much for themselves as possible. Sometimes it may seem easier to complete the task yourself. However, in the long run, time will be saved when the care recipient is able to complete simple tasks.

A person with mobility problems is at great risk for falls. A decrease in muscle strength and flexibility, along with changes in vision and hearing, are two of the reasons for this increased risk. Falls are the leading cause of injury-related fatality among older adults. Many falls can be prevented through following regular exercise programs, having regular vision and hearing check-ups, and making the home a safe place to live.

A FALL PREVENTION PLAN

Falls are a common problem among older adults. Most falls occur in the home. There are several things that you and your loved one can do to reduce the likelihood of falling.

Some fall prevention strategies have already been discussed. Here are some important points to remember.

- Maintain a regular exercise program to improve physical strength.
- Have the doctor review the medications that may be causing dizziness or balance.

- Limit alcohol; it only takes a small amount to make a person feel off balance.
- Make sure your loved one gets up slowly from a sitting or lying position to prevent dizziness.
- Wear proper-fitting shoes with low heels and a nonskid sole.
- Check the feet for such problems as corns, bunions, and ingrown toenails.
- Make certain your loved one knows how to use the walker or cane if needed for walking.

The home environment may also pose a problem for an older adult with mobility problems. Hazards within the home can actually make a mobile person immobile and cause falls. A few basic changes can make your home a safer place.

In the Living Areas

- Make sure that all rooms have good lighting.
- Remove scatter rugs.
- Remove electrical cords and telephone wires from walking paths.
- Arrange the furniture so that walkways are free of clutter.
- Ensure that telephones are easily reached, not attached to the wall.
- Put handrails along both sides of stairways, and light switches at the top and bottom of each stairway.

In the Bathroom

- Install night lights.
- Install grab bars near the tub, toilet, and shower.
- Use nonskid rugs in the bathroom and a rubber-suction mat in the tub.

You cannot prevent all falls, but a few changes in your home environment may help reduce the risk of falling. U.S. Consumer Product Safety Commission (800-638-2772) has more information about home safety. They can also send you a free copy of their booklet, the *Home Safety Checklist for Older Consumers.*

WHAT TO DO IN CASE OF A FALL

Even the most attentive caregiver will not be able to prevent all falls. For that reason, you need to know what to do in case a fall does occur.

If someone falls, the first thing to do is to check and make sure that the person is awake and alert. Reassure the person while you check for any injuries. Do not try to move the person by yourself. This may actually be more harmful. If there is an injury, call the emergency services, usually 911. Be prepared to give them the person's name, address, telephone number, and condition. Stay with the person until the ambulance arrives.

If there are no injuries and the person can get up with a little assistance, help them to a chair. Don't try to lift the person by yourself. Wait for help! Whether there is an injury or not, it is always important to let the doctor know about the fall and what may have caused the fall. For example, dizziness may be caused by a new medication or a heart problem. If the person who has fallen becomes confused or complains of persistent pain, you need to contact their doctor for an evaluation.

Falls do occur in the home. However, you now know how to prevent them, and you are prepared to respond, if the situation arises.

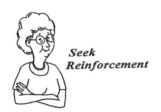
Seek Reinforcement

Remember, you are not alone as a caregiver. There are many resources, like your doctor, nurse, or physical therapist, who can provide you with the necessary information you need to care for someone at home. There are also support groups for caregivers. Contact your local senior center or the Alzheimer's Association for more information. Also check the list of additional resources listed in the appendix of this book.

Caregiving is not an easy task. So remember to reward yourself daily for the goals you have achieved. If you think positively, get the information you need, and seek reinforcement, you will be able to deal with the joys and challenges of caregiving. You can do it!

Here are some questions to help you review the information discussed in this chapter:

1. What are some points to remember about good body mechanics?
2. What self-care activities can you do to prevent a back injury?
3. What are some exercises that can improve strength and flexibility?
4. What are the benefits of exercise?
5. Name five problems associated with immobility.
6. Name five things you can do to help prevent falls.

7

Bathing and Dressing

Patricia Edwards, Shelia Collier, and Cornelia Beck

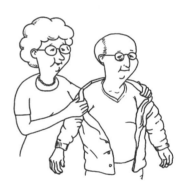

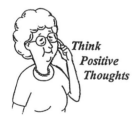

*Think
Positive
Thoughts*

I have a friend named Rose. She is the caregiver for her husband, Roy. Recently, Rose asked if I could help her find someone to assist with Roy's morning. I asked Rose if she needed someone to bathe and dress her husband. Rose said, "No, I do not want someone to bathe and dress Roy—I want someone to help Roy bathe and dress himself."

I have thought many times of Rose's wisdom. Rose realized the importance of Roy maintaining as much independence as possible, yet Rose had the wisdom to take care of herself by asking for some help.

If you are a caregiver like Rose, you probably know that helping someone bathe and dress can be time-consuming and tiring. Therefore, you must take time out to take care of yourself before you can effectively take care of someone else.

Be gentle with yourself. You didn't create all of the problems you face daily, but you are coping and meeting daily demands as best you can. However, realize that you will meet those demands better on some days than on others. Just like the person for whom you are caring, you, too, will have both good and bad days. Again, be gentle with yourself on the "bad days."

Establish a routine schedule when you take time out. Rose wanted to schedule her time out when someone came to assist Roy with bathing and dressing himself. Rose was wise in choosing this particular time of the day for her time out because, as we age, morning often becomes the peak time for our energy level. Therefore, Rose might be more inclined to do things for herself during the morning when she has the energy.

Rose planned to use this time to have her coffee, read the paper, exercise, and on nice days walk outside. Rose thought that if she managed her time effectively, she could accomplish these enjoyable activities while someone helped Roy bathe and dress himself. Rose's plan sounds wonderful, especially the exercise because it can be very effective tool to reduce stress.

If you also care for a family member who needs help bathing and dressing, you'll probably agree that this is a good time to accept some help, whether it be 2 or 5 days a week. Therefore, making a list of helpful resources available to you is probably an important step toward reaching your goal.

When making a list of resources, use your imagination, and be creative. It is easy to feel alone and overwhelmed when faced with being a caregiver. Most people think of only the obvious sources, such as children and grandchildren. However, many times children and grandchildren have career and family demands that will not permit them to be available for hours when people normally think of bathing and dressing. Although bathing and dressing seem like sequential activities, the bathing could occur the night before, making dressing in the morning less time-consuming. If you can allow yourself the flexibility of bathing the night before, perhaps your resources could include children and grandchildren.

Rose could afford to pay someone to assist her. However, many times older adults living on fixed incomes cannot afford this service. Perhaps children or grandchildren who have careers might contribute by paying someone to assist, which brings us to another major point: *Do not be afraid to ask for help.* Even if the person you asked is not able to help you in the manner you requested, this person may have some good alternatives for helping you in your caregiving endeavors. Keep an open mind to all offers of help.

Although family may be the first avenue of assistance, also remember neighbors and church friends. Another good source is the local Area Agency on Aging. This organization will send a social worker to your home, and together you and the social worker can determine services to receive. Many times people are eligible to have home health aides to assist with bathing and dressing. As the primary caregiver, you will direct the care and decide how bathing and dressing occurs. So let's discuss some of the ways that Rose and you can plan bathing and dressing activities. Remember that you are planning these activities for yourself, as well as for the person for whom you are providing care.

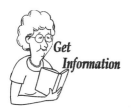
Get
Information

By now you have made a list of your resources and have decided to be gentle with yourself and to take good care of yourself. Now you are going to gather information to help with in the activities of bathing and dressing. Don't feel overwhelmed at the prospect of information gathering because you probably already have more information than you realize. As a matter of fact, if you are the primary caregiver, you probably have more information than anyone else. Whether the care recipient has experienced changes in physical capacity, mental capacity, or both, the person probably continues to have the same daily preferences. Let's use Rose and Roy as an example. Rose knows that Roy always drinks his coffee before bathing and getting dressed in the mornings. More than likely, neither physical nor cognitive decline has changed this preference. Therefore, Rose will provide more consistency for Roy if she permits him to drink his coffee before bathing. If Roy's daily routine is continued, Roy may feel more secure, confident, and motivated to participate in daily activities.

To some extent, we are all creatures of habit. In this phase of information gathering, take a few minutes to reflect and recall the routine, habits, and preferences of the person receiving care. You may even want to list those habits and preferences to periodically check whether you are addressing those preferences.

BATHING

Along with feeling clean, bathing is a great way to relax and rinse tension away. Nothing feels as good as being clean. Think about the times when you took that warm bath and got into bed between clean sheets. That feeling is one of the most comforting things you will give. Providing a bath is a wonderful opportunity for you to be creative. For instance, Rose knows that Roy has always enjoyed listening to soothing music. Therefore, Rose might play soothing music during Roy's bathing routine.

Water is one of the healing wonders of life. Water turned into bathing becomes a very comforting experience. You will have the opportunity to create a soothing and relaxing mood so that the bathing experience will be a reward all by itself. Perhaps you may think of various ways to decorate your bathroom for this relaxing experience. Use flowers or candles to create a soothing atmosphere during bathing. Bathing results in increased self-esteem and feelings of well-being. My grandmother was my grandfather's caregiver after he had a stroke. I have fond memories of my grandfather as clean, shaved, and smelling a little like "Old Spice."

During the aging process, people may lose certain physical or mental functions that had enabled them to maintain and direct their own bath or personal hygiene. Or they may have retained certain functions and need minimal help with bathing. You, as the caregiver, need to determine the level of assistance required. Regardless of the amount of help needed, try to arrange for the care recipient to have a private, warm, and soothing bath.

PURPOSE AND TYPES OF BATH

The purpose, type, and frequency of the bath depend on the condition and bathing preferences of the care recipient. Just as Rose knows Roy's bathing preferences, you probably are already aware of the previous bathing patterns of the person for whom you are caring. Therefore, you may need to spend some time reflecting about ways to best meet those preferences.

You will need to look at the reason for giving the bath. The purpose of bathing helps determine the frequency and type of bath to give. Some reasons for bathing include preventing infection by removing germs, providing warmth, eliminating odors, increasing activity, or promoting relaxation.

Baths range from showers, tub baths, sponge baths, and partial baths to complete bed baths. Special baths, such as the "towel bath" keep the skin free of lesions and cuts, and are gentle and soothing, especially for the elderly. A lot of effort has been put into developing products for bathing and skin care. Therefore, you will have a variety of products from which to choose. When choosing products for bathing the older adult, remember that the skin should remain clean and dry. Bathing every day with dry harsh products or without rinsing well may lead to skin problems.

Give complete sponge baths in bed to individuals who cannot move well or at all, such as the person who has had a stroke. Acquire a hospital bed, and place a trapeze bar over the hospital bed. The trapeze bar helps the person move so that you may wash body parts more easily. The bar also helps the caregiver when changing the sheets. If used properly, the trapeze bar enables the person to get more exercise and perhaps maintain some upper body strength. My grandfather had several strokes and needed complete bed baths until he regained the use of one side of his body. I remember the day my father placed a trapeze bar over my grandfather's bed. The bar helped him to move better and get stronger. As he continued to gain strength, he could wash most of his body parts and required help with only a partial bath.

The partial bath is for persons who can do parts of their own bathing but need help with other parts. People with mobility or strength problems benefit from partial baths. For instance, the person who has had a stroke may be able to reach most body parts but may need help to reach others, such as feet and legs. This type of partial sponge bath often occurs in the bathroom near the sink.

Showers and tub baths are ideal for persons with the mobility to get into and out of the shower or tub without hurting themselves. However, persons receiving shower and tub baths may still need supervision. For instance, Roy can walk with assistance, so Rose purchased a special chair, which she can move from the tub to the shower. Roy sits on the chair whether he is bathing in the shower or in the tub. By using this chair, Roy does not get so tired while bathing. This decreases the possibility that Roy might fall in the shower or tub. If the chair sounds like something that might work for you, please check to see whether your insurance will pay for the chair. Remember those resources and ask for help!

Whirlpools are great when they are available. If you have access to a whirlpool, it provides a relaxing and invigorating bath. Check on eligibility for physical therapy because a physical therapist may offer an occasional whirlpool bath.

Towel baths help keep a person warm and relaxed in bed with moist warm towels covering the body. This type of bath helps people who need to rest, are immobile, need warmth, or just need a change from the regular bathing routine. To give a towel bath, moisten large towels with a warm no-rinse soap solution. Move the towels while keeping the body covered with a blanket over the towels.

A relaxing massage using lotion can top off all types of baths. Massaging with gentle lotion helps preserve healthy skin and prevent skin breakdown. Remember to remove excess lotion from the skin and avoid any type of harsh lotion. Special lotion is available for elderly skin.

Safety is of utmost importance. Avoid bath oils that make the tub slippery, and install nonskid stickers and grab bars because most falls and injuries occur in the bathroom. The person receiving care may need to use a walker, a hearing aid, glasses, or other assistive devices. Replace these devices as soon as possible if you removed them during the bath.

When you can, offer choices about bathing. Ask such questions as: "Do you want to take a bath or a shower?" Offering the wash cloth, you might also ask: "Would you like to help wash?"

You may need to ask yourself some of the following questions: Can the person I am caring for move well enough to reach and clean all body parts? Is he or she mentally and physically able to carry out parts of bathing? How much and what type of help is needed to bathe and dress? What other persons or devices do I need to complete the bath for my care recipient?

BATHING THE CONFUSED PERSON

If you are bathing a person with Alzheimer's or another type of dementia, speak slowly, keep eye contact, and finish one thing before moving on to the next task. You may need to break up the bath to avoid tiring the person. For instance, you may choose to bathe the upper portion of the body, rest, and then bathe the lower portions of the body.

It is especially helpful for someone familiar to take care of the person with confusion. You will want to use some of the following techniques to keep the confused person from becoming agitated, uncooperative, or angry. Avoid asking the person to do tasks that are too difficult to understand or do. Avoid too much noise and activity. Remember that it is easier to prevent agitation than to try to deal with it once it occurs.

If the confused person resists taking a bath "right now," wait and return to bathing later. If the bath is for routine cleanliness, you may do it later. However, if the person is incontinent of urine and bowel movements, try to bathe as soon as possible to prevent skin breakdown. You might offer a complete bath and a comfortable massage, or you may clean just the area that needs cleaning.

HOW OFTEN TO BATHE

Most older adults do not bathe themselves every day. Their skin tends to get dry, and excess bathing may make it even drier. How often to bathe depends on individual needs. You may choose to use different types of baths in 1 week. You may decide on a tub bath once a week and partial baths as needed in between.

Home Care for Older Adults: A Guide

What are some general things to remember about bathing? Knowing the reason for the bath, the type of bath, and how often to bathe creates a routine pattern for you. Family and friends who are caregivers of those they have known for a long time have an advantage because they already may know what the person likes and dislikes.

Skin breakdown is a serious problem for older people. Rings, fingernails, and other sharp objects can easily tear their skin. You will want to look for any red or irritated areas during the bath and report this to the nurse or physician. Start with the cleanest parts of the body first (face, neck) and work your way toward the less clean areas (rectum, genitalia). When using a bath basin, change at least once and more often if needed. Avoid rubbing the skin dry. Pat the skin dry with a towel to prevent skin breakdown. Handle skin with great care because a break in the skin offers a way for infection and other problems to occur.

Make sure you remember to include privacy during bathing. Have the bath water and towels ready before you begin. Let the person touch the water to check the comfort of the temperature.

Give instructions and make verbal, facial, or physical gestures slowly. Giving specific verbal instructions, one at a time, will help increase communication and eliminate surprises. Wait until the end to wash the face and shampoo the hair. Or you can do as Rose does. Rose makes shampooing a separate activity to prevent Roy from getting too tired. If the person is confined to the bed, use a shampoo board or an inflatable shampoo basin. The inflatable basin is more comfortable.

Some older adults may only take partial baths. I visited a 92-year-old woman who took a sponge bath every day, had her hair done once a week at the beauty salon, and always appeared (smelled) clean. She had decided that it was very dangerous for her to get into a shower or bathtub, but she could do her partial bath just fine. Some older adults may want to stand in the shower with their walker and a chair behind them for extra safety precautions. No two persons will take a bath exactly the same way.

Most people enjoy doing for themselves as long as possible. Therefore, encourage the care receiver to continue to do as much as possible. As Rose often says, "The key is to keep moving." Your most important role as a caregiver may be to encourage as much self-care as possible and create fun ways to keep moving.

I hope that the bathing tips we have discussed will be helpful to you. Remember, just keep trying until you find what works best. When you find something that works, *share* the information with other caregivers. You will find it helpful to network with other caregivers and share successful, and not so successful, ideas and strategies on bathing and dressing. However, before I discuss specific dressing information or strategies, let us review some of the points you need to remember as a caregiver.

- Take care of yourself.
- Take time out to take care of yourself.
- Be gentle with yourself—you did not create all of the problems you face daily. You will do your best, realizing that "your best" may vary from day to day.
- Exercise to relieve stress.
- Do not be afraid to ask for help.
- Make a list of all resources. Use your imagination and be creative.
- Look for strengths, not just weaknesses; if you only look for the weaknesses, you will never identify the strengths.
- Allow yourself to be flexible—there is usually more than one way to do what has to be done!

DRESSING

As people age, there are many reasons why they might need assistance in dressing. Older adults who have conditions, such as arthritis and Parkinson's disease, may have physical limitations that make dressing a challenge, whereas the older adult with Alzheimer's disease may have cognitive or mental challenges to independent dressing. Whatever the challenge, mental or physical, look for the strengths. Remember that people are unique and have different strengths and weaknesses.

After you have identified what the person receiving care can do, you may be able to make changes in the environment to help more independent functioning. For example, if the person has arthritis, he or she may experience problems with buttoning and zipping and tying shoes. However, if you've provided garments and shoes that have Velcro instead of buttons, zippers, or shoe strings, the person may be able to do much of the dressing independently. Although not all problems and solutions are as simple as providing Velcro, for almost *every* dressing challenge there are some ways to make the experience easier. I will discuss some ways, but there can be others. If the ways discussed are not helpful to you, do not give up. Remember that every person and every situation is unique. The ways that might work best for you may very well be the unique ones that you discover yourself.

INVOLVE THE CARE RECEIVER IN DRESSING

Think about past patterns of dressing. Did the person receiving care choose his or her own clothing each morning—or did someone else? If he or she has always selected clothing each day, this pattern should continue to the extent that it is possible. Letting individuals choose their own clothing serves several purposes. Choosing clothing promotes a sense of control. Being able to make a small choice is important for self-esteem because many other choices, such as driving, cooking, gardening, or traveling, may no longer be possible.

If the person receiving care has dementia, he or she may not be able to choose appropriate clothing. However, you can still try to use dressing as a means of letting the person make choices. Instead of opening the closet door and letting the person choose from "everything" in the closet, *you* can put out a few things—like two sweaters or two shirts and two pairs of trousers that match and are appropriate. By giving the person the opportunity to exercise some control, you may be increasing self-esteem, motivation, and decision making.

As you gather information and formulate plans, think about the expression "Use it or lose it." Rose and I spoke about the expression as it related to Roy. We discussed that if Roy did not use his mental and cognitive processes to make decisions, he would lose the ability to do so. If Roy did not *use* his ability to move his arms through the sleeves of his shirt, he would soon experience changes in his muscles and joints and *lose* the ability to do so. If Roy had Alzheimer's disease and did not *use* his ability to perform habitual tasks like dressing, he would soon *lose* his ability to do so. Therefore, Rose knew how important it was for Roy to continue to do as much for himself as he possibly could.

Again, I thought about Rose's wisdom in understanding the importance of self-care for Roy. Many times you, the caregiver, may feel that it is cruel to force the care receiver to do as much as possible. That feeling, as well as the feeling that you can dress the person faster by yourself, may lead you to providing total care during dressing. Thus, the dependent person soon loses the ability to participate in dressing. With that loss can come decreased self-esteem, frustration, depression, and decreased cognitive and physical functioning.

While gathering information and formulating a plan for dressing, remember that you, the caregiver, are largely responsible for the interaction that occurs during dressing. If you are stressed, rushed, or frustrated, the person you are caring for may sense this and become acutely aware of his or her increased dependency, and dressing will become unpleasant.

How to Make Dressing Easier

Try to use a calm, relaxed, unhurried manner. Remember that most of the responsibility for the interaction during dressing rests with you. If you, like Rose, are planning to take your time out while a home health aide is doing the bathing and dressing, plan to be present with the new caregiver the first 3 or 4 times. It will give you time to teach the new caregiver the strategies that work best for you. Although you need to remain open to ideas and strategies that a new caregiver may have, the new caregiver also needs to be willing to use those strategies that have worked for you.

Dressing a Person Who Has Physical Limitations

Dressing is almost mechanical because people dress so often over a long period. Therefore, nearly all people retain some ability to dress themselves. As we stated earlier, people with physical limitations will experience different challenges to dressing than will people who have mental or cognitive limitations. Therefore, not all interventions are appropriate for everyone. You must select those strategies

appropriate for your situation. In other words, identify the strengths
and limitations. Then you will select the appropriate type of assistance that is needed.

For people with physical limitations, some tips for successful
dressing follow:

- If one side of the body is stiff or does not "work as well" as
  the other side, put on and take off clothes from the stiffer side
  first.
- If standing balance is affected, the care receiver can sit on the
  edge of the bed or in a chair with armrests to dress.
- Use loose, lightweight clothing (jogging suits are great).
- Use elastic waistbands or velcro closures instead of buttons or
  zippers.
- If the person can raise his or her arms, use pullover tops to
  eliminate fastening.
- If the care receiver has problems raising his or her arms over
  the head, choose clothing that closes in the front.
- Use elastic shoe laces or slip-on shoes.
- Put shoes on with a long-handled shoehorn.

DRESSING A PERSON WHO IS CONFUSED

If you are caring for a person who is confused and unable to communicate verbally, it is difficult to know the dressing preferences of
the person. You may need to use trial and error to find out what will
work best. Don't be discouraged if something works one day but
seems to fail the next day. Many times people with dementia have
emotions that they cannot verbally express. With your patience, your
consistency, and the person's successful achievement of some of
the activity, the buildup of negative emotions may decrease.

Again, remember that the caregiver sets the tone for the dressing
experience by the initial approach to the situation. Tell the person
what to expect, such as: "You are going to get dressed." Keep your
conversation simple. Give one direction at a time. The following
are tips for independent dressing:

- Speak slowly, clearly, and succinctly. Avoid shouting.
- Use one- or two-step commands. For instance, say: "Put on your socks" instead of "Put on your clothes." An example of a one-step command is: "Put your leg in the pants." A two-step command would be "Stand up, and pull your pants up." You will have to determine whether the person can follow two-step commands.
- State instructions in a positive manner. Tell the person what you *want* done, not what you *don't want* done. For example, say "Put on your shoe," instead of "Don't take off your sock."
- Make statements instead of asking questions. For example, if you ask, "Can you button your shirt?" you may get a negative response. Instead say, "Button your shirt."
- Repeat commands with a calm voice, eye contact, and a positive attitude. Give the person plenty of time to follow your instruction before repeating them.

Remember, each individual is unique, and the same things do not work for everyone. If physical guidance fails, try modeling or gesturing. For example, Rose might point to Roy's sweater, pick up the arm of the sweater, point to Roy's arm, and then point back to the arm of the sweater. If gesturing proved unsuccessful, Rose might pick up her own sweater and put her arm through the sleeve. Then she would hand Roy his sweater and guide his arm to the sleeve. This is an example of modeling.

If the person is easily distracted, change the environment to keep him or her focused on dressing. Control the noise level. The television or the radio may be a distraction. The room should be at a comfortable temperature. None of us can focus well if we are uncomfortable. Rule out other that which could interfere with making appropriate choices, such as visual problems. Arrange light-colored clothes against a dark-colored bedspread for contrast. Remember to lay out only appropriate choices of clothing.

Rose tries to anticipate and plan ahead to meet Roy's needs. She tries to control Roy's choices. Most of the time Roy selects his clothes from the choices that Rose has provided. However, sometimes Roy becomes agitated when trying to select what he will wear. On such days, Rose tries to limit the decisions Roy has to make. She does this by making selections for Roy. However, Rose still encourages Roy to participate in dressing by placing Roy's clothes in the order that he will wear them. This is called sequencing. By doing this, Roy does not have to remember which item to put on next.

REWARDING SUCCESSES

To be successful, the person you are caring for does not have to completely dress alone. Even a small increase in the person's participation counts as a success. Remain flexible in judging successes and failures. Rose knew the importance of rewarding Roy for his efforts. Rose knew that Roy loved to eat chocolate chip cookies. Because Roy was not a diabetic, Rose served him a chocolate chip cookie after dressing. She knew that he also appreciated verbal praise for his efforts. Therefore, Rose told Roy how well he had done in bathing and dressing and how proud she was of his efforts.

Some people may enjoy a trip outdoors, whereas some, like Roy, may prefer a favorite food as a treat. However, just a word of caution in determining what reward or reinforcement to use. Avoid using activities, such as favorite television or radio programs, as rewards because these activities are ones that the person you are caring for may be able to enjoy every day. Limit rewards to those things that do not restrict other enjoyable daily activities.

REINFORCEMENT

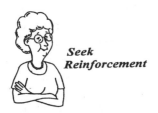

Seek Reinforcement

I have discussed the idea of reinforcement for the care receiver. When Rose gave Roy chocolate chip cookies for participating in dressing, that was reinforcement for Roy. Now let's discuss reinforcement for you, the caregiver! It is just as important for you to reward yourself as it is to provide reinforcement for the person for whom you are caring. Make a list of the various ways to treat yourself. Whatever you like to do, keep trying and planning until it becomes a reality. You also could join a support group for caregivers like yourself. If you don't know of any caregiver support groups, try calling your local hospital and asking for a social worker to assist you in finding such a group. Talking with other caregivers can help relieve stress, and it also is a means of exchanging ideas and tips.

As I mentioned in the beginning of this chapter, you must be gentle with yourself. You will have both good and bad days. Some days the person may resist your help. Avoid interpreting this as failure. It does not mean that you did anything wrong. It simply means that what you tried did not work that day. You have limitations as everyone else does.

Remember, you must take care of yourself. Follow good nutrition, exercise, rest routines, and take time out for yourself. Follow Rose's example. Reward yourself for being wise enough to ask for and accept help! If you, first, follow these suggestions for taking care of yourself and, second, follow the suggestions for bathing and dressing, you and the person you are caring for will benefit.

8

Staying Healthy—Eating Right

Jane Campbell

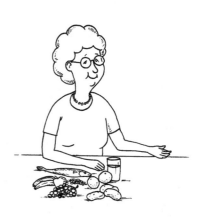

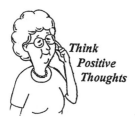

Think Positive Thoughts

Have you ever heard the expression "You are what you eat"? Your eating habits are influenced by your cultural background, your family ties, your role in society, and how you are feeling. Family traditions are linked to food, and the way it is cooked, served, and eaten. As we grow older, good eating habits can become a much more important matter.

The best-seller book *Chicken Soup for the Soul* reminded me of my mother who thought chicken soup was the answer for everything when you were sick. As a child, if I had the flu or any ailment that my mother thought was worthy of her home-made chicken soup, she would cook up a big pot, and I was expected to eat it all. To this day, when I am sick, I remember my mother making chicken soup and being convinced it would make me well. Today many people, including nutritionists, present evidence that chicken soup may indeed have healing properties. Other foods are also being identified that can have a negative effect on our lifestyle and will be discussed at a later time in the chapter.

In addition to getting nutrition, mealtime is a time for socialization. Advertisements often show families gathered around a dinner table or couples sharing a meal with flowers and an intimate atmosphere. An atmosphere needs to be created at a mealtime that encourages us to eat well and digest our food easily. Playing music, putting fresh flowers or candles on the table, or having family and friends over to share a meal can often help us to eat so much better. These kinds of things are also important to the person you are caring for and perhaps needs to be fed.

Mealtime can be a lonely time, particularly after the death of a spouse or companion, with whom an older person shared many meals. Well-balanced, inexpensive meals and socialization are often available at community senior centers and day care centers. You might want to check on what is available for you or your dependent older adult.

NORMAL AGING CHANGES AFFECTING NUTRITION

As we grow older, there are some normal aging changes that affect our nutrition and health. For instance, older adults may become less active, and their metabolism slows down. Thus, we burn less calories than younger people. Growing older, however, is not an excuse for gaining extra pounds. We need to watch what we eat and keep our weight within the given range for our height and age rather than allowing pounds to add up over time. Making wise food choices is important for the health of all ages, but it is even more important for older adults, particularly for older adults with chronic health problems. Not eating foods with the needed nutrients leads to malnutrition, a common problem among older adults. Nutrition is further threatened because the body's ability to absorb nutrients declines with age. Many older adults also take several medications, which interfere with the absorption of nutrients and appetite.

Another normal aging change is that the tongue loses some of its taste buds. Food that was once flavorful may taste bland and unappealing. However, the ability to sense bitter tastes does not decrease. The combination of bland and bitter may result in an unpleasant, metallic taste in the mouth. As taste becomes a little "duller," many people try more and more salt and sugar to improve the flavor of foods. A healthier alternative is to add flavor with herbs and spices, such as garlic, onion, rosemary, oregano, thyme, cinnamon, and nutmeg.

Aging also brings about changes in the gums. This does not mean that older adults need to lose their teeth. Teeth loss is not a normal aging change but is usually the result of gum disease and the lack of preventive dental hygiene. Seeing a dentist on a regular basis and practicing good oral hygiene can help prevent loss of teeth for many older adults. It is an important aspect of caregiving.

Changes also occur in the salivary glands, so that the older person has a small decrease of saliva in the mouth. For the most part, the dry mouth that older adults often get is a result of center drugs they are taking. Good oral care needs to include regular brushing after meals, flossing of teeth at least daily, and regular check-up by a dentist.

Difficulty swallowing is another problem found with aging. The esophagus, the tube between the mouth and the stomach, does not push the food down into the stomach as well as it use to. Also, the valve at the end of the esophagus does not close as tightly. Food can back up from the stomach into the esophagus, causing an unpleasant feeling of fullness, indigestion, or burning and pain. The result can be less pleasure and more discomfort when eating meals.

There may also be a decrease in the stomach or gastric juices, which impairs digestion and absorption of some of our vitamins and minerals, such as iron, vitamin B_{12}, and protein. The bowel, known as the large intestine or colon, is frequently a cause for concern among older adults. The bowel does play a role in digestion and is important as a storage organ. Age can cause shrinking of the lining of the bowel and a decrease in muscle tone. Some anal, rectal changes are due to a loss of muscle elasticity. It is often difficult to determine if the changes in the bowel are caused by aging or a decrease in activity, a lack of fiber in diets, or the side effects from medications. Changes in bowel habits or color of stool are a need for concern and should be reported to the physician or nurse.

DIET AND NUTRITION

It is just as much a problem to eat too much food as it is to not eat enough of the right food. Excessive body weight stresses the heart, muscles, and bone. It increases the likelihood of hernias, hemorrhoids, gallbladder disease, and varicose veins. It can aggravate arthritis and other chronic conditions. A healthy diet (low fat, low calorie, and high fiber) combined with exercise reduces your risk of numerous health problems, such as cancer, heart disease, stroke, osteoporosis, and diabetes. Eating right helps you control overweight complications and other health problems, such as elevated blood sugar, blood pressure, and cholesterol levels. Good eating also improves energy level, moods, and how you feel about your appearance. Eating in healthier ways usually means deciding to change and then doing it slowly. One way is to learn more about what a healthy diet includes (see Figure 8.1).

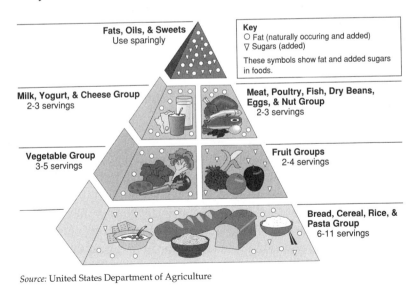

Source: United States Department of Agriculture

FIGURE 8.1 *Food guide pyramid*—**a guide to daily food choices.**

The goal of a healthy diet is to eat a wide range of foods every day from each of the major food groups: the bread, cereal, rice, and pasta group; the vegetable group; the fruit group; the milk, yogurt; and cheese group; and the meat, poultry, fish, and dry beans, eggs, and nuts group. Stay away from foods that are high in fat and sugar. They provide calories but not the nutrients you need. Eat lots of beans (kidney, pinto, lima, etc.) Beans are an excellent nonfat source of carbohydrates, fiber, vitamins, and protein. Choose 1% or nonfat milk.

FOOD PLANNING

No single diet or food plan is right for everyone. Mass advertising promotes high-profit processed foods and soft drinks, promising fun and eternal youth but delivering only empty calories. Stores are now beginning to provide more varieties of ethnic foods and new foods that can improve our food selections. Healthy unprocessed foods can be flavorful and interesting. The old expression, "an apple a day keeps the doctor away" holds true for all ages.

For many people the kind of food they eat is influenced by the cost. Some suggestion for a limited budget include buy only as much as you can use or store, and buy the unprocessed foods that give you the most nutrition per dollar. Examples are low-fat cottage cheese, dried beans, chicken, protein-enriched spaghetti products, peanut butter, oatmeal, low-fat milk, whole-grain cereal, and catfish or other inexpensive fish. Frozen vegetables are often less expensive than fresh and have approximately the same nutritional value. Fresh seasonal fruits are good, such as apples, oranges, and bananas, and have higher nutritional content than canned fruits, which are often much higher in sugar content because of the processing.

The manufacturers are now required to label the food packaged in the United States with information about the recommended daily allowances for certain nutrients, calories, fat content both saturated and unsaturated, and the other nutrient information. At times it can be confusing to read all of the labels, but with practice and guidance, it will help you to develop a good food plan. In choosing your foods, you need to consider the carbohydrate, protein, and fat content as well as the vitamins and minerals.

CARBOHYDRATES

Carbohydrates are the sugars and starches you eat. As your body grows older, the ability to digest large amounts of sugars decreases; therefore, your blood sugar climbs higher after eating sugar than when you were younger. Although this does not mean you should avoid sugar and sweets entirely, you do need to eat sweets in moderation. Carbohydrates are a ready source of energy and, therefore, are a very important part of your diet. Carbohydrates should provide 60% or more of the energy needs for older adults and for brain functioning. Adequate carbohydrates intake keeps the body from using protein as an energy source, so that protein can be saved for rebuilding and restoring cells that become damaged or destroyed.

PROTEINS

Proteins should supply 15% or more of your daily requirements. Proteins are the building block of your body. Proteins are important for all growth and development. As you grow older, they are very important for repairing and rebuilding tissue all over the body. Proteins are found in all meat and fish as well as in dairy products, such as milk, eggs, and cheese. The soybean plant is also a good source of protein.

FATS

Some fat in the diet is good for your health, but, unfortunately, most people eat too much of it. Americans have a higher fat content in their diets than most other people in the world. Fats should be less than 30% of your daily diet. Fats are part of the basic structure of every cell. Fats furnish twice as many calories per gram as carbohydrates and protein in your diet. Fats act as carriers for fat-soluble vitamins (A, D, E, and K) and provide insulation and protection for our organs and the skeleton. Excessive dietary fat can contribute to aging and certain diseases, such as coronary artery disease, atherosclerosis (hardening of the arteries), and cancer. There is especially strong evidence in the link between dietary fat and colon cancer. Avoid eating large amounts of foods high in fat content, such as eggs, butter, and whole milk, and animal fats, such as red meat. To cut back on your fat intake, try grains and beans or legumes instead of animal protein whenever possible. Fish and skinless poultry are animal proteins that are lower in fats. When you eat red meat, use leaner cuts. Try to use nonfat dairy products or reduced fat products available. Substitute fresh vegetables and fruits or low-fat yogurts for snacks instead of potato chips or cookies. Use cooking oils sparingly, and choose those lowest in saturated fat and cholesterol, such as canola, corn oil, olive, or sesame. Try preparing your food in ways other than frying, such as steaming, grilling, or baking. Avoid buying foods with more than 3 grams of fat per 100 calories. Remember to read the labels.

CHOLESTEROL

Cholesterol is a fatlike substance found in the bloodstream. High levels of cholesterol are found in coronary artery disease. Too much cholesterol can be related to heredity, eating patterns, or cultural preferences. There is both "good" and "bad" cholesterol. High-density lipoprotein—or the good cholesterol—has a protective effect, but low-density lipoprotein—or the bad cholesterol—is linked with coronary artery disease.

WATER

Water is not a nutrient, but it is an important element for life and is often overlooked in a food plan. Our bodies are made mostly of water, which is vital to maintain life and health. Water is essential for proper functioning of our kidneys and bowels. It helps to transport nutrients and medications to the body and helps to get rid of body wastes. As you age, your body does not control your fluid balance as well. Drinking 6 to 8 glasses of water each day becomes very important. Water can also be obtained from soups, juices, beverages, fruits, and vegetables. Coffee and other beverages containing caffeine actually push fluids out of your system and should be avoided.

FIBER

A high-fiber diet (one that has a variety of whole grains, fruits, beans, and vegetables) helps to prevent constipation, reduce risk of colon cancer, diverticulitis, and other illnesses. Studies also indicate it helps lower cholesterol and reduces your risk of heart disease. Fiber helps to hold water, providing the soft bulk that absorbs body waste. As a result, fiber helps our bowels work more smoothly. This is important as you grow older and your bowel loses some of its elasticity and mobility, which can increase the tendency toward constipation. Different forms of fiber have different functions: For example, oat bran is thought to lower cholesterol, whereas wheat bran does not. Pectin from apples and beans prevents diarrhea and helps excrete cholesterol. Fiber does have its negative side, in that a high-fiber intake can cause gas and bloating. It can also interfere with calcium, iron, and zinc absorption. A wise course is to have enough fiber (and adequate fluid intake) to make your bowel movements soft and easily passed. It is important to avoid the use of laxatives and other medications that stimulate the colon unless recommended by your physician.

A good food plan can be done on a limited budget. Often it is difficult for a single person to prepare food and not have leftovers. A great way to handle leftover vegetables is to place any of them in containers after your meal. Put the container in the freezer, when it is full you will have a great base for a pot of vegetable soup. A good food plan can save money by keeping you healthier and avoiding costly medical bills than can result from poor nutrition. A good food plan that includes well-balanced meals contains enough vitamins and minerals in the food you eat. It is usually not necessary to purchase supplemental vitamins and minerals if you are eating well. It is a good idea to discuss the need for a daily vitamin pill with your physician or nurse before you decide to take them on your own.

FOOD AND DRUG REACTIONS

You need to be cautious when taking any vitamin or mineral supplements, as they can have a negative effect on your body. All medications, both over-the-counter and prescribed drugs, as well as herbal or "home remedies," can affect the body's response to the action of other drugs you take. Over-the-counter drugs do not require a prescription, but they can have just as many side effects as prescription drugs. The response of our bodies to medication changes over the years; in later life, the body becomes more sensitive to chemicals and drugs. It is important that you read and follow the direction on all medications. Check with your pharmacist about any questions you may have about your medications. Because your body's ability to control fluid balance does not work as well in the older adult, taking adequate fluids with medications is important. You need to remember the following three Ws: What is it?; Why do I need it?; and When do I take it? In addition, how long should you take it? It is never good to practice to stop taking any medication before it is all gone unless you talk with your physician or nurse first. If a medication causes you any discomfort, or if you develop a reaction of some type, call your physician immediately and report it. It is very easy to forget to take your medication no matter what your age. Establishing a plan for taking your medication at the same time every day or having a certain routine can help you in remembering to take your medications. For those who take multiple drugs, there are special medication holders sold at drug stores that can serve as a reminder for whether or not you took your medications.

Older adults, particularly the frail elderly, who are on multiple prescription medications for chronic conditions, need to have their drugs followed closely. Several drugs can contribute to poor appetite and eating problems. Sometimes more than one drug can have an affect on the loss of some nutrients, creating a serious deficiency. An example of this might be a potassium deficiency caused by the use of both diuretics and laxatives. Some drugs can affect the metabolism, absorption, and excretion of foods and drugs. The level of the medication in the bloodstream may go higher than is desirable. Your pharmacist can give you information about how your specific medications and food interact with each other.

As I mentioned earlier in the chapter, fluids also play an important role in drug absorption. Ice water can delay the dissolution of capsules. The practice of taking medications with very little fluid is not uncommon for older adults and as a result may cause a delay in the absorption of the medication. The age-related decrease in stomach acids can impair the absorption of calcium and iron as well as certain drugs used as antidepressants. Emotional stress can delay the emptying time of the stomach and create problems with medications, particularly antibiotics and heart medications (see Table 8.1).

TABLE 8.1 Specific Drug Effects[a]

Drug	Effect
Over the counter	
Aspirin	Iron loss
Antacids	Phosphate loss, thiamine deficiency
Laxatives	Decrease in potassium, calcium, magnesium, zinc, vitamins, A, D, and E
Prescription	
Antibiotics	Can decrease riboflavin, vitamin C, and calcium absorption and destroy the bacteria in the intestinal tract that produces vitamin K
Phenytoin (Dilantin)	Decreases vitamins, D, K, and folic acid
Phenobarbital	Decreases vitamin D
Indomethacin (Indolin) and other anti-inflammatory drugs	Iron loss
Chlorpromazine hydrochloride (Thorazine) and Thioridazine (Mellaril) Tricyclic antidepressants	Decrease in riboflavin, weight gain or loss

[a]These are only a few of the common drugs that can affect nutrient absorption in older adults. Check with your pharmacist for any other medications that could have a drug-nutrient effect.

MANAGING FEEDING PROBLEMS

DENTAL CARE

Good mouth care is an important part of staying healthy and eating right. Tooth pain and sore mouth can sap your energy and cause distress for weeks and months at a time. Tooth loss can prevent you from eating well if soft nutritious foods cannot be substituted for those that can no longer be chewed. To try and keep your teeth healthy, remember these rules.

- Brush your teeth after you eat.
- Floss daily.
- Eat well-balanced meals and drink water.
- Schedule dental check-ups at least once a year.

Tooth loss does not have to be a natural part of aging. It is important when you brush your teeth to do it correctly. Ideally, it would be good to brush after every time you eat, but it should be done at the very least daily. The preferred method is to use a brush with soft rounded, nylon bristles, keeping the brush at a 45-degree angle against the gumline. Wiggle it in a circular motion and then away from the gum. When brushing your teeth do not forget the tongue because bacteria collect on the tongue and spread to the teeth. After brushing, rinse the mouth with warm water and floss between all the teeth. A clean mouth will stimulate appetite and food will have more appeal.

DENTURES

Unfortunately, it has been in only recent years that the importance of dental care has been heavily emphasized. Medicare covers our health needs, but it does not include dental care. For people who wear dentures, soaking is never enough; it is important to brush them with a soft brush using a commercial powder, paste, or hand soap. Weight loss, especially for older adults with dentures, can trigger certain oral problems. For instance, loose-fitting dentures can cause sores and open areas in the mouth, and the chewing process becomes painful.

As a result, some may avoid foods that require much chewing, such as meats, which is a valuable source of protein. Substituting products that are not as difficult to chew but are a good source of protein is helpful. Soybean products, cheeses, and eggs are good sources of protein that can be prepared and eaten without too much problem. In addition, a blender can be used to chop up or puree the food that is more difficult to chew. It is important to look in the mouth when an older person complains of some discomfort in the mouth. Use a flashlight to check for any redness or open areas in the mouth. It is important to get a dental check-up whenever you suspect problems with the proper fit of the dentures. A person who has dentures needs to wear them regularly. The shape of the mouth will start to change if dentures are not worn. Denture adhesives are not very effective and should be used for a limited time only. The dentures often will still wiggle even with the adhesive and cut the mouth and interfere with chewing. It is good to have dentures relined when they start to slip instead of trying to make them fit with glue.

MEMORY PROBLEMS AND EATING

Changes in eating patterns often occur, if one is experiencing memory loss. A person with memory loss may forget to eat. Safety must also be considered. Stoves and electrical appliances may be left on accidentally. Close monitoring or removal of an appliance that can create a safety hazard should be considered.

A person with memory loss is at higher risk for choking on food. When the muscles in the mouth and throat do not work together to move the food from the front of the tongue to the back of the throat and begin to trigger the swallow, food is often tucked away in the jaws. You need to encourage the person with memory loss to chew and swallow the food. Taking too large a piece of food and not adequately chewing it before swallowing may cause it to lodge in the throat. A caregiver can take steps to prevent this from happening by cutting the food into smaller bites or putting food in a blender to chop it.

Dry foods, such as cake or bread, can also cause problems. As you recall from earlier in the chapter, the amount of saliva for older persons decreases, and mouths are drier. Using water or other thin liquids to "wash down" any food is risky and can also cause aspiration or choking. To try and prevent this from happening here are several tips.

- Have the person sit up as straight as possible.
- Avoid tilting the head back and extending the neck.
- Have the chin tilted downward and slightly forward.
- Encourage coughing if foods gets caught in the throat.
- Observe the dependent person during meals if swallowing is a problem.

In the event that the person you are caring for actually begins to choke, remain calm and ask, "Can you speak?" If the person cannot respond, then you need to do the Heimlich maneuver. If you are not familiar with doing this, you could contact the American Red Cross for information and classes on the Heimlich maneuver.

WEIGHT LOSS

One of the most common ways to determine if a person is eating enough is to check the weight. Weigh at the same time of day and with the same amount of clothes. Keep a record of the weight, and a record of food intake. If there is a weight loss of 10 lb or more within 6 months, bring that information to the attention of the physician or nurse. A nutritional supplement may be needed. Special formulas available in supermarkets have all the nutrients needed for a balanced diet. One of the commonest supplements that is advertised is Ensure. There are many other brands available. Check with the physician or nurse about the best supplement for your particular situation.

TUBE FEEDINGS

If the person receiving your care is no longer able to eat or maintain adequate nutrition by mouth, the physician may suggest a feeding tube. The feeding tube can be placed into the stomach. Managing feeding tubes can be a challenge for caregivers. You need to make sure that the person is sitting up during the feeding to prevent the fluids from going into the lungs. Signs of aspiration or fluid in the lungs are coughing, choking, difficulty breathing, increased rapid breathing, gurgling voice quality, or change in skin color. Sometimes a person can "silently aspirate," and it is not detected by the caregiver. If the person begins to have frequent episodes of pneumonia, it may be the result of silent aspiration of liquids. There needs to be further evaluation and follow-up by a physician. Another key concern with feeding tubes is clogging of feeding tubes. Flushing the tube with about an ounce of warm water before and after the tube feeding can usually prevent clogging. Diarrhea may also be experienced with tube feedings. Although not everyone develops this problem, it is not unusual if it does happen.

You also need to closely watch the feeding to be sure the formula does not spoil. Most tube-feeding formulas are in cans and can be stored in the cupboard. If only a portion of the feeding from the can is used, the rest of the feeding needs to be refrigerated until it is ready to be used again. For tube feedings that are given continuously by means of a feeding pump, formula should not hang for more than 8 to 10 hours before it is changed, or the bag is rinsed with water and more feeding added. The home health nurse will provide you with information and education on how to prepare tube feedings and what to watch for to prevent problems.

WHAT YOU CAN DO

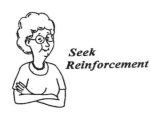

Seek Reinforcement

Remember that age-related changes can have an influence on older adults' eating patterns and their health.

Two major age-related changes that effect nutrition are altered metabolism (way the body uses the food) and changes in digestive functions of the stomach and bowel. Medications may also influence a person's ability to meet the bodies need for essential nutrients. The following are key points for the caregiver to remember.

As you review your eating and dietary habits, you should ask these questions.

1. Do you read the food guide pyramids available on many of the cereal products and try to eat a wide range of foods every day from each group?
2. Do you need to reduce your overall fat intake, such as cutting down on processed meats (i.e., cold cuts and lunch meats and deep-fried foods)?
3. Do you substitute high-fat snack foods, such as chips and pastries, for foods lower in saturated fat?
4. Have you reduced your sugar and salt intake?

Good eating habits along with exercise and a desire for a healthy lifestyle can make a difference in how you feel about yourself.

As a part of *Healthy People 2000*, a national effort is being made to provide nutritional screening for adults older than the age of 65. The *National Nutritional Screening Initiative* is an effort supported by national associations of dietitians, physicians and nurses. The "Determine Your Health Screening Tool" has been widely distributed to older adults through the senior center system, senior advocacy groups, and health care providers. The tool can be used to identify older adults who are at risk for poor nutrition and who could develop health problems as a result. You can contact any senior center in your area and obtain additional information about the program.

9

Bowel and Bladder Problems

Susan Sherman

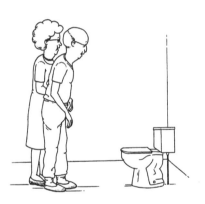

One of the more troublesome situations a caregiver may face is the start of a urine or bowel problem. Probably about 99% of the time, the problem involves the bladder only. Occasionally, it will involve both the bladder and bowel.

Although these problems can be unpleasant to deal with, part of the reason they are unpleasant is our lack of knowledge and perhaps negative feelings we learned as we were growing up. Think for a moment about the emphasis placed on "potty training" or the shame a child feels when they have an "accident." Think about the slang words related to basic bowel and bladder function that have such negative meanings. We have some of the feelings and beliefs because we do not really understand how our body functions.

Although the main purpose of this chapter is to help you manage urinary or bowel problems effectively, the first hurdle is simply thinking about the problem and talking about it. Here is some important information to remember.

We know incontinence is not a part of normal aging. Therefore, you need to talk with the physician and nurse about the problem and help them look for the cause. Incontinence should not have to be the "straw that broke the camel's back." Ask for a referral if your physician is unable to help you. Many treatments for incontinence do not involve surgery. You are not alone in your concern about this problem. Surround yourself with a team of health professionals, who can help you work through these problems. Your positive outlook is so important.

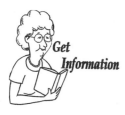

Get
Information

This chapter discusses basic aging changes and how to recognize and manage urinary and bowel problems. Medicines and medical problems affecting the bowel and bladder, nutrition and hygiene considerations, and establishment of routines are also covered. Although some older individuals experience bowel and urinary problems together, the information for these problems is presented separately.

URINARY PROBLEMS

Whenever older people experience urinary problems or symptoms, they should speak with their doctor or nurse about them. It is common to feel some embarrassment about starting a discussion about urinary problems. It may help to know that many people are having the same or similar problems and are seeking help for it. In fact, nearly one half of all elderly being cared for at home experience some type of urinary problem, particularly uncontrolled urine leakage (also called urinary incontinence). The information you receive about incontinence problems will help you to talk about it more easily. Urinary problems are really no different from other symptoms that we report to the physician or nurse. The following chart includes terms often used to discuss urinary problems. You want to become familiar with them.

1. *Urinary incontinence*—accidental leakage of urine.
2. *Urinary frequency*—a need to go to the bathroom very often, usually eliminating only small amounts of urine at a time.
3. *Urgency*—getting very little warning about the need to urinate; unable to hold urine for 10 to 15 minutes after the first urge to urinate is felt.
4. *Urge incontinence*—accidental loss of a large amount of urine closely following the "urge" sensation.
5. *Stress incontinence*—accidental loss of urine with activities, such as coughing, sneezing, laughing, or lifting.
6. *Retention*—difficulty getting all the urine out of the bladder.
7. *Nocturia*—getting up during the night to urinate.
8. *Dysuria*—pain with urination.
9. *Prolapse*—a condition in which the bladder or bowel itself protrudes into the vaginal area.
10. *Overflow incontinence*—a condition in which the bladder overflows with urine, the urine is not emptying completely, and the urine continuously leaks out (occurs with prostate enlargement (blockage) or with damage to the nervous system as with stroke).

Urinary incontinence or urine leakage is the most frequently reported symptom that older individuals experience. Other symptoms are often reported along with the leakage.

AGING CHANGES THAT CAN ALTER URINARY ELIMINATION

You might find it helpful to refer to Figure 9.1 as you read this information. The bladder is the part of our body that has the job of holding our urine or water and is located in the lower part of our

URINARY SYSTEM

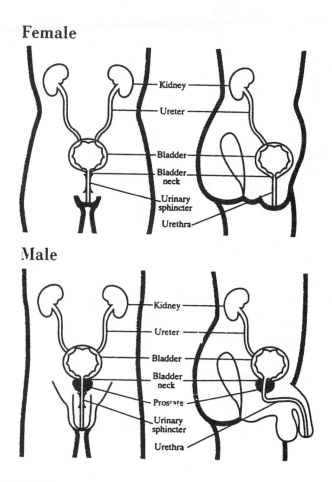

FIGURE 9.1 Urinary system.

abdomen. Urine is simply water plus other substances that our kidneys have filtered out. The water and other substances are not needed by the body. Even though urine may normally have a slight odor, it is really a clean substance that does not have germs (or microorganisms) in it. Urine is normally a pale yellow color. It is not normal to have blood or other particles in urine.

As we age, some of the changes in our urinary system may affect the way our urinary tract works. It is important to keep in mind that basic aging changes do not necessarily lead to problems for everyone. Leakage of urine does not occur simply because someone is old. A reason for the problem can usually be identified, and, in many cases, it can be treated in a way that improves or eliminates the condition or changes the way we are responding to it.

As we age, the kidney becc ;es a little less efficient in filtering things not needed from the body. It is also believed that blood flow to the kidney is slower during the day than it is at night. The increased urine production at night results in the need to go to the toilet during the night. Anyone who is getting up to the bathroom two or more times during the night needs to have the problem checked.

Aging changes cause the bladder to become smaller, so that the bladder holds smaller amounts of urine. If there have been repeated infections over the years, the outlet of the bladder can become narrowed and lead to urination difficulties. In addition, the muscles that support the bladder on the pelvic floor (this is the very bottom of the body's trunk) may have been weakened by childbirth, surgeries, or generally poor physical conditioning. This muscle weakness has been identified as a contributor to stress incontinence where small amounts of urine leak when a person coughs, sneezes, or laughs.

Sensation of how much urine is in the bladder may also change with age. When we are younger, we have a sensation when the bladder is about one-half full. When we are older, we may not get that sensation until the bladder is very full. As a result, the bladder may be prepared to contract and empty very soon. If we are prevented from getting to the toilet quickly, which might happen with arthritis of the knees or hips, an incontinence episode can occur.

Only men have a prostate gland. The prostate gland lies around the small tube from the bladder, the urethra. With advancing age, the prostate slowly enlarges. For many men, this poses no problem whatsoever. However, for some the enlarging gland pushes on that small tube, the urethra, making it more difficult for urine to pass. Think of the difficulty you would have blowing bubbles through a straw if you pinched it off a bit with your fingers. You have to push harder to get the air past the barrier. If prostate enlargement begins to push on the urethra, it becomes more difficult for the older man to push urine past that barrier. The stream of urine will become smaller and less forceful. Some individuals will have difficulty starting to urinate. This is called hesitancy. After the man has finished urinating, dribbling of urine may occur. When these symptoms are noticed, it is important to seek an evaluation. Leaving these symptoms unevaluated over years can lead to chronic infection and overfilling of the bladder, which can result in more serious problems.

The most important change that occurs for women only is the loss of estrogen associated primarily with menopause. This can also happen with surgical removal of the ovaries (some hysterectomies include removal of ovaries) or other medical treatments. When women's estrogen levels get low after menopause, the tissues inside the urethra (that small tube leading from the bladder to the outside) weaken and do not close as well. As a result, leakage of small amounts of urine may occur. Another result of this estrogen change may be a condition known as an "unstable bladder." An unstable bladder results in frequency and urgency, or urge incontinence. The doctor may order an estrogen supplement if hormones are the suspected cause of urinary problems.

CHANGES IN PHYSICAL AND SOCIAL ENVIRONMENTS

Although we cannot say that physical and social factors are real aging changes, they are so important for the elderly that they should always be included in this kind of discussion. As aging progresses, many older adults are less able to meet the demands of their home environment. For example, they may have difficulty going up and down stairs, they may not be safe alone because of instability, and they may not be able to run the vacuum sweeper or a snow blower to clear the walk. They may spend a great deal of time in the kitchen during the day, but the toilet is on the upstairs level or on the other side of the house. For an older woman with urinary urgency, this may be the difference between being wet or being dry.

It is very helpful to check the home environment. Is the bathroom close enough to where the person usually spends his or her time? In addition to distance, are there stairs to climb, and is the lighting adequate? Is the toilet the proper height, and are there grab bars available to steady oneself while sitting down? Is there adequate privacy if others live in the home?

The social environment refers to the other persons around the older adults, persons who live with the older adult, and people in the community. Is someone available to help the older adult to the bathroom if necessary or empty a commode pail or a urinal? These critical factors can spell success or failure for the individual.

MEDICAL PROBLEMS CONTRIBUTING TO INCONTINENCE PROBLEMS

It is always helpful to clarify whether the urinary incontinence or other symptom is a problem that has just started or has been a problem for a long time. Symptoms that develop suddenly require immediate attention from the physician. Let us take a look at some of these acute or sudden-onset problems.

Urinary Tract Infections

A urinary tract infection can lead to incontinence that had previously not existed. *Always notify the physician for burning or pain sensation during urination, urgency, frequency, cloudy or bloody urine, fever, or chills.* Other complaints may include lower back pain, which is relieved after urinating. An examination of a urine sample will show whether there is an infection.

Infection of the Vagina or Urethra

Infections of the vagina (birth canal) or the urethra (tube leading from the bladder to the outside of the body) can lead to incontinence. Symptoms may include frequency, pain with urination (dysuria), or urgency. A physical examination will confirm whether or not this is the problem. This condition is uncomfortable, but is easily treated by the physician.

Bowel or Fecal Impaction

A bowel or fecal impaction is the presence of hard, dry stool in the bowel. It is believed that this mass presses on the bowel and, in turn, presses on the bladder. When the impaction is removed, continence is usually restored. The best treatment for bowel or fecal impaction is prevention. Prevention is best accomplished by adequate fluids and fiber in the diet and daily exercise.

Diabetes

Elevated sugar levels in the body can produce large amounts of urine and irritate tissues in the pelvic area, increasing the risk of infection. If the bladder does not empty, it becomes very large and overfilled. Small amounts may leak out of the bladder.

Neurologic Disorders

Incontinence can be the result of neurologic diseases, such as Alzheimer's, Parkinson's disease, stroke (also called cerebral vascular accident) and multiple sclerosis (MS). The most common problems seen with these diseases is the inability of the bladder opening to relax completely to allow the flow of urine. When the bladder is overly full of urine, a constant dribbling of urine will occur. If you are caring for someone who has experienced a stroke or who has Parkinson's disease or MS, be sure to ask the physician to evaluate their urinary system, especially if they experience continuous dribbling of urine.

With a disease, such as Alzheimer's, the sufferer can empty the bladder completely but may not remember where to go for toileting, how to remove clothing, or how to ask for help. These individuals are best helped using the techniques listed under the scheduled toileting program.

Delirium and depression are other conditions that may be associated with incontinence. These conditions are discussed in Chapter 4.

MEDICATIONS THAT CAN CONTRIBUTE TO INCONTINENCE PROBLEMS

Because each medication cannot be listed individually, a general rule of thumb is to check with the physician to find out if a certain medicine or medicines can be causing a urinary problem. Here is a list of the most common groups of medications that may cause urinary problems.

Diuretics—remove extra water from the body.

Sedatives—may cause drowsiness and decrease the awareness of sensations of bladder fullness.

Pain medicines—may cause drowsiness and decrease the awareness of sensations of bladder fullness.

Heart or blood pressure medicines—may either cause overrelaxation of bladder muscles or lead to the retention or holding of extra urine.

Antidepressants—may cause sedation and secondarily affect toileting urges; these medicines cause sedation, which decreases response to these medicines and can also prevent the bladder from emptying.

Alcohol—may lead to symptoms of urgency, frequency, and sedation and may make it difficult to get to a toilet in time.

There are many other groups of medicines used less frequently with older adults that can have an affect on bladder problems. If bladder problems occur, you will need to check with the doctor to find out whether any of the medicines may be contributing to the problem.

RECOGNIZING AND MANAGING URINARY PROBLEMS

Many people feel they are experiencing urinary problems because they are not as young as they used to be. The first important question to ask is, "Is this a new problem?" If this is a new problem, it may be the result of some of the conditions we've already discussed. The physician needs to be called. Many of these conditions can be treated successfully after an evaluation. If treatment does not take care of the problem, this condition may be chronic, meaning that it is continuing over a long period. Because many older adults hide incontinence problems from family (even spouses), you may not have been aware of an ongoing problem. Many caregivers suspect a problem from stains on clothing or furniture.

For chronic cases of incontinence, it is important for you, the caregiver, to ask the physician whether a referral to a continence specialist would be possible. Chronic incontinence is treatable. There are several options available. As a first step, you can begin gathering information about the problem with a bladder diary. Take several sheets of paper with lines and make columns (draw lines to make four columns) and headings as in Table 9.1. It does not have to be typed. You will probably need more rows than shown here.

In the section labeled *day/date,* just insert that information. Starting at the same time every day, use the bladder diary for 2 or 3 days. Each time you enter information, be sure to include the time. Under *time and amount/fluids taken,* write in the time and what the person drank and how much, such as "7 a.m., water, ½ cup" or 7 a.m., prune juice, 1 cup." Then, "7:30 a.m., decaf coffee, 1 cup." Then under *time and amount of urine* you would enter "8:15 a.m., small amount" or "8:15 a.m., large amount." Estimating the amount as small, medium, or large is fine. Under *leakage/amount,* you would record the amount of urine that leaked out before the dependent older adult made it to the toilet. In the column, *reason/leakage,* write what led to the leakage. For example, if a coughing spell led to a small amount of leakage, you would write that in.

It would be ideal if the person you are caring for is able to help you with this. If not, you will have to keep track the best you can. It is helpful to write down as much detail as possible. This record can help your physician or continence specialist figure out what may be leading to the problem. You may even come to some conclusions on your own. For example, you may discover that the person receiving care is having fewer or more incontinence episodes than you had thought. You may also discover that he or she is not drinking enough

TABLE 9.1 Bladder Diary

Day/date	Time and amount/ fluids taken	Time and amount of urine	Leakage/ amount	Reason/ leakage
Monday, May 12	7 a.m. water ½ cup 7:30 a.m. Coffee, 1 cup	8:15 a.m. Large amount	Small	Coughed

fluids (less than 6–8 glasses a day). Many people think that drinking less fluid will lessen leaking. Not true! Taking less fluid can actually lead to an increase in leakage because the urine becomes concentrated. Remember the following general tips when considering a toileting problem:

- Make sure chairs have arms and are easy to get out of.
- Make sure that the height of the chair is correct for the person using it. Feet should rest comfortably on floor when sitting with the back against the backrest.
- Check to see whether the person can easily get up out of the bed and that the bed is not too high.
- Provide an assistive device (a cane or walker) if that is needed to get to the bathroom. Training from a physical therapist may be needed.
- Remember the benefits of exercise to improve mobility skills and general conditioning.
- Make sure that the clothing you provide is easy to get off and on.
- If the person demonstrates difficulty walking, inspect the condition of the feet, including the length of nails and the presence of painful foot conditions, such as bunions or other pressure areas.

The following are specific bathroom tips to promote toileting independence:

- Toilet seats should be at appropriate heights. If the person has hip problems, a raised toilet seat may allow greater comfort using the toilet.
- Grab bars can provide the added support an older person needs to raise up from the toilet seat.
- Use urinals as needed.
- Use commode chairs as needed; make sure chair is stable and not easily tipped over.
- Check on getting adaptive devices that make safe transfer from wheelchair to toilet possible.

- Keep bathroom private, well lit, and warm, with secure scatter rugs on the floor.
- Use toilet paper that is fragrance free; it is less irritating.

PROVIDING PHYSICAL ASSISTANCE TO THE TOILET

Taking the time and patience to begin toileting on a schedule and providing the physical assistance to get to the toilet is all that is needed to stay dry. Research has shown that many nursing home patients regain their continence when they are physically assisted to the toilet every 2 hours (see the Scheduled Toileting Program later). For an elder who is confined to a wheelchair, this schedule may still be possible. It will be necessary to learn how to transfer to the toilet and back to the chair safely. The physical therapist or home health nurse can provide this instruction.

NOCTURIA OR URINATING DURING THE NIGHT

If a person is having difficulty with frequent urination at night, you may want to try restricting the fluids taken after 6 in the evening. Frequently, this restriction is just enough to cut down on trips to the bathroom during the night. Sometimes, noise or pain also can awaken the person.

Provide a night light or put a flashlight at the bedside for use when getting up to toilet. Instruct the person to sit up on the side of the bed for just a few seconds before walking to the bathroom, just so they can "get their bearings." If mobility or balance is a problem, you can provide a urinal or bedpan right next to or in the bed or position a bedside commode chair next to the bed. A word of caution on the use of these items is in order. Some older adults will feel very ashamed and embarrassed by these items. As the caregiver, it is helpful for you to explore how the person feels about them.

KEGEL EXERCISE OR PELVIC MUSCLE EXERCISES OR BIOFEEDBACK

These exercises are prescribed for various types of urinary incontinence. They are simple to learn and perform, but they should really be supervised by a continence specialist or nurse who has had special training. If the exercises are not being performed correctly, no progress will be made. If exercises are performed in the wrong way, they can actually worsen symptoms. This treatment is an excellent choice, however, especially if the incontinent person is able to follow simple instructions and is motivated. These exercises are usually not helpful for persons with dementia.

PROVIDING INCONTINENCE PRODUCTS

Many products are available to assist keeping a person dry. Older adults, especially frail elders, need encouragement. There are so many beliefs and feelings involved that careful, sensitive attention is necessary. Elders have reported that they feel like children, are filled with shame, experience embarrassment, and so on, simply because of incontinence.

Pads, diapers, and reusable undergarments are popular ways of handling the wetness associated with incontinence. Pads and diapers range from minipads to large layered diapers. These products should be considered only for long-term use after a careful evaluation of the incontinence has been completed. They should be carefully chosen based on need. The home health nurse can help you make choices or tell you where to go to find out about the products.

GETTING HELP

Contact your local hospital or home health agency for assistance. You may ask for a nurse who specializes in urology, continence, geriatrics, or wound and skin. Another resource to check with is a durable medical equipment company. Sometimes that can even be your local pharmacy. They may have people available to help you choose products that would do the best job for the particular level of a problem. There are several national organizations dedicated to problems of incontinence. These organizations are the National Association for Continence and the Simon Foundation. Their addresses are included in the appendix of this book.

Use of products like catheters, condom catheters, and the like is really beyond the scope of this chapter. If you are caring for a person who needs these items or is currently using these items, they should be receiving care and supervision by a physician and a home health nurse. Unapproved use of these products can have serious consequences.

FOODS THAT CAN CONTRIBUTE TO URINARY PROBLEMS

There are several foods and liquids that can potentially affect urine control. The following list of foods and beverages includes those items that can lead to symptoms, such as urinary urgency and frequency for certain people:

- Coffee (this includes decaffeinated coffee)
- Tea
- Alcoholic beverages
- Carbonated beverages
- Soft drinks with caffeine
- Milk and related products
- Medicine that has caffeine as an ingredient
- Citrus juices and citrus fruit
- Tomatoes and tomato-based products
- Sugar, honey, and corn syrup
- Artificial sweetener and any drinks using artificial sweetener
- Chocolate

Some medications will lead to a change in urine color, particularly some used to treat urinary problems. If the urine has changed color following a change in medicines, check with the pharmacist. The medication is probably the cause. If the urine has a strong odor and is darker in color, it usually means that the person has not had enough to drink, and the urine is concentrated. This is a problem because it can lead to a urinary tract infection. If there are no other unusual symptoms, make sure you give fluids right away. If there are symptoms, such as urgency, frequency, pain, or any of the other symptoms discussed earlier, the doctor should be called because a urinary tract infection may have developed.

RECOMMENDED FLUIDS AND FOODS

Taking adequate amounts of fluid is the simplest measure to promote good urinary elimination and general health. Unless the physician has recommended limited fluid intake, 6 and 8 glasses of water are recommended daily. A very easy way to assure fluid intake is to fill a 2-quart pitcher with water every morning, place it in the refrigerator, and make sure that it is finished by the end of the day.

The best beverage to drink is water. However, many persons do not care for water. Adding just a small twist of lemon can help improve the taste of water for many. Juices that cause no problems are apple, apricot, cherry, cranberry, grape, and pear and prune. Also, several herbal teas are available that can be used as a substitute for regular teas and coffee.

In addition to fluids, foods high in fiber help promote full emptying of the bowel. As mentioned earlier, an impacted bowel can lead to urinary incontinence. Bran is an excellent source of fiber that many elders find helpful in maintaining regularity. In fact, there are several high-fiber supplements you can make at home that will help with regular bowel movements. With the extra fiber, you will need to make sure the person is taking in enough fluid. You can use this recipe instead of some of the higher-priced supplements found in the pharmacy. Remember that the addition of a high-fiber supplement may initially cause some bloating and gas, but as body adjusts these problems will decrease. The following is a special fiber supplement recipe:

1 cup applesauce
1 cup bran cereal, crushed (or unprocessed bran)
½ cup prune juice
Dash of cinnamon or nutmeg (for flavor)

Mix ingredients. Keep refrigerated in a clean covered container.

When starting the fiber supplement begin taking 1 to 2 tablespoons with a large glass of water. This can be increased up to 8 tablespoons per day to achieve a soft bowel movement.

ESTABLISHING A ROUTINE SCHEDULE FOR ELIMINATION

When an older adult is having urinary symptoms, it is often helpful to establish a routine for urination. If you worked on the bladder diary in the earlier section, you may have discovered that the person is going to the toilet every hour. People sometimes do this in an effort to avoid an accident. If this is the case, these are tips that you can follow for the problem of urinary frequency:

- Make sure that irritating foods or fluids are not being taken.
- Make sure fluid intake is about 6 to 8 glasses of fluid daily.
- If the person is not taking an adequate amount of fluid, gradually increase the amount until the body adjusts to the increase.
- Gradually lengthen the time until using the toilet. If he or she is going every hour, initially have the person wait an hour and 15 to 30 minutes, then 2 hours, and so on. Every week, lengthen the time interval until it reaches 3½ to 4 hours.
- If the person feels the urge to go to the bathroom before the time is up, ask him or her to follow these steps to decrease the urge to urinate.

1. Relax and focus on breathing in and out deeply.
2. Tighten muscles in the pelvic area as if to hold back gas and then relax them.
3. Wait a few minutes, and then go on to the bathroom.

If the person you are caring for has a demanding illness and is experiencing confusion, it is likely that you will not be able to follow the steps outlined previously. What you can do, however, is place the person on a scheduled voiding program, assisting him or her to the bathroom every 2 hours. Scheduled toileting has been shown to reduce the number of incontinent episodes. Follow this program.

- Assist the person to the toilet first thing in the morning.
- Ask the person to empty his or her bladder completely.
- Praise him or her for urinating in the toilet.
- Offer fluids at this time.
- Toilet the person every 2 hours.

- Ask the person to let you know if he or she needs to go before 2 hours.
- Follow up every 2 hours, providing praise and encouragement for maintaining dryness.
- Keep a log of his or her progress.

PRODUCTS THAT MAY HELP WITH EITHER BLADDER
OR BOWEL PROBLEMS

Products included here are items that you can purchase at the local pharmacy, durable medical equipment store, or discount store or by mail order. First and foremost, check with your physician or nurse to find out which products will be useful. You do not want to waste money on products that will not serve your needs. Also, check with your physician or seller to find out whether the product would be covered by your insurance plan. Some products that can be used for incontinence appear in Figure 9.2.

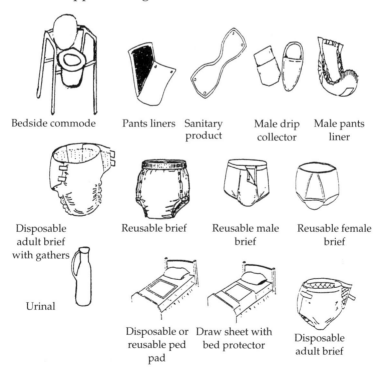

FIGURE 9.2 Incontinence products.

BOWEL PROBLEMS

The purpose of this section is to acquaint you with information that can help you provide care for a person experiencing bowel difficulties. The broad areas that will be covered are basic aging changes related to the gastrointestinal (GI) system, medical problems and medicines that can lead to or aggravate an existing bowel problem, nutrition and hygiene issues, and routines for elimination.

Bowel problems are quite common among the elderly. The three main problems in this discussion are constipation, diarrhea, and bowel or fecal incontinence. Fecal incontinence is much less common than either constipation or diarrhea. As a medical condition it is relatively harmless. Fecal incontinence is much less common than urinary incontinence. It is included for discussion because it can be devastating for the individual experiencing it and difficult for the caregiver.

A definition of common terms is included to help you understand and communicate with your physician and other health care professionals with more confidence and ease. Bowel problems, like urinary problems, can create barriers to communication because of the embarrassment and shame that is felt when talking about such issues. Knowing the terms and what they mean can help overcome that difficulty so that problems can be addressed and solved. Here are some definitions.

1. *Constipation*—there may be a feeling of fullness, pressure in the rectum, abdominal or back pain, and lack of appetite, then straining and the passing of dry, hard stool or a decrease in the frequency of stools.
2. *Fecal impaction*—hard mass of stool lodged in the colon or rectum.
3. *Diarrhea*—frequent passage of loose, fluid-informed stool.
4. *Fecal (bowel) incontinence*—involuntary or uncontrolled passage of stool soiling bed, clothes, chair, or floor.
5. *Peristalsis*—rhythmic movement of the large intestine, which results in the "pushing" or removal of stool from the rectum.

Aging Changes That Can Alter Bowel Elimination

To talk about aging changes that affect bowel elimination, we need to talk about all the organs of the GI system (see Figure 9.3). The purpose of the GI system is to take in nutrition in the form of food and fluids for the body and break it down into some form the body can use. We take food into our mouths, chew it up, and mix in with saliva, which helps the chewing action and prepares food to be digested.

Once food gets into the stomach, various fluids are secreted to further prepare the food for our body to use. It moves through the small intestine, then through the large intestine. The small and large intestines are able to contract to move the digesting food along. As contents move along, fluids and nutrients are absorbed. The final product, the bowel movement or stool, is delivered to the rectum. Generally, the nerves in the rectum are stimulated by stool present and that is when the urge to have a bowel movement occurs. The muscles of the rectum contract, and stool is expelled, helped along in part, by gravity.

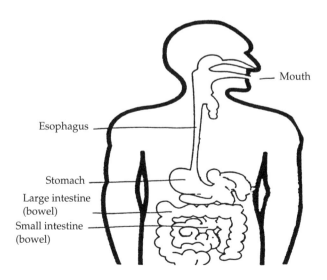

FIGURE 9.3 Organs of the gastrointestinal (GI) system.

Passage of the food through the entire system can normally take up to 5 days. The usual or normal number of stools for an individual varies a great deal. Most adults have a bowel movement in the range of two in a single day up to once every 3 days. It is helpful to remember, however, that bowel function can be affected by diet and fluid intake, exercise, time of day, and even the environment. The presence of fiber in the diet can lessen the amount of time it takes for food to pass through.

I briefly describe each part of the GI system and the aging changes that may eventually affect bowel elimination.

Changes in the Mouth and the Esophagus (Tube to the Stomach)

The aging process contributes to slight changes in the mouth and esophagus related to food and digestion. Gums often recede. However, with good oral hygiene, this change does not have a big effect on the function of the mouth. Also, some areas of the mouth that produce saliva decrease their function, but overall there is adequate saliva production. Changes in the mouth and esophagus that cause problems with chewing and swallowing often result from disease (such as stroke), the use of medication, or poor mouth care. The person may develop such problems as loss of teeth, loss of taste, or dryness of the mouth.

Changes in the Stomach

The major aging change seen in the stomach is a decrease in the ability to produce the hydrochloric acid that breaks down or digests certain foods. The decrease in acid production may be due mainly to a change in the mucous lining of the stomach.

Changes in the Small Intestine

Researchers remain uncertain about the actual aging effects on the small intestine. It is believed that there may be a decrease in the amount of area needed to absorb nutrients, but it is still not proven. It is known that vitamin A absorption is improved in the elderly, but that vitamin D and calcium may not be absorbed as well.

Changes in the Large Intestine

It is believed that changes in the blood vessels that serve the large intestine may undergo changes that result in less blood flow. It is thought that the ability of the large intestine to move is also affected by aging.

MEDICAL PROBLEMS THAT CAN CONTRIBUTE TO BOWEL PROBLEMS

Diseases That Can Lead to Chronic Confusion

Diseases, such as Alzheimer's disease, Multiinfarct dementia (small strokes), Parkinson's disease, and other diseases that are caused from damage within the central nervous system, frequently lead to constipation and fecal incontinence.

Diarrheal Illness

Many common illnesses can lead to diarrhea including influenza, bacterial infection, food intolerance, diabetes, inflammatory bowel disease, and malnutrition, to mention just a few. Diarrhea can become serious. Because stool is moving rapidly through the GI tract, the nutrients needed by the body cannot be absorbed properly. Loss of fluids also poses a threat. Contact should be made with the physician to find out what to do. Because of the possible side effects of over the counter medicines, they should not be given without physician consultation.

Another condition that masks itself as diarrhea is fecal impaction. The mass or the impaction itself causes the large intestine to produce mucus. Bacterial activity is also stimulated. As a result, a foul-smelling brown liquid begins to pass around the fecal mass. This is frequently mislabeled as "diarrhea." If treatment for diarrhea is given, the condition can worsen. Removal of an impaction is important, the home health nurse can perform the necessary treatments.

It is extremely helpful for the caregiver to consult with the physician ahead of time about what over-the-counter medicines to use for common problems, such as diarrhea, headache, and constipation. The reason this is so important is that many problems can develop when mixing various medications and even with mixing medications with certain foods.

Poor Function of the Rectal Sphincter

The rectal sphincter is the small band of muscles that help close off the rectum. You squeeze these muscles if you need to stop the passage of gas or stool. When a problem exists either physically with the sphincter or the person cannot control the sphincter, problems maintaining continence can develop. Physical damage to these muscles can occur from Crohn's disease, diabetes, radiation treatments, to name a few. The loss of sensation of the rectal sphincter can be caused by stroke, tumors, and alteration in sensation caused by drugs, such as sedatives.

MEDICATIONS THAT CAN CONTRIBUTE TO BOWEL PROBLEMS

Antacids

Antacids that contain magnesium as an ingredient can cause diarrhea.

Antibiotics

Antibiotics can lead to diarrhea because the normal "good" bacteria that live in the bowel and help break food down as part of digestion can be sensitive to the antibiotic being given. When these "good" bacteria are also destroyed, stool will pass more quickly through the GI tract. When diarrhea is occurring with antibiotic therapy, it is frequently helpful to give products that contain lactobacillus (Lactinex), yogurt (with active cultures), or buttermilk because either have bacteria cultures that help replace the friendly bacteria being destroyed.

Laxatives

Rather than simply relieving constipation, laxative use can lead to diarrhea. Laxative use is believed to be excessive among older adults. With frequent use, many laxatives can become habit forming because the body begins to rely on the drug for cues about emptying the bowel rather than responding to the natural cues that signal movement of the bowels. One popular laxative mineral oil reduces the absorption of vitamins A, D, E, and K. It may also interact with other drugs, such as anticoagulants.

Tranquilizers and Smooth Muscle Relaxants

These classes of medication can lead to problems with constipation by decreasing muscle movement in the large intestines.

RECOGNIZING AND MANAGING BOWEL PROBLEMS

Constipation

Older people can have several factors that contribute to having a problem with constipation. Constipation is a health problem leading many elderly people to be mistaken about the belief that they must "clean themselves out" on a regular basis to avoid future problems. These beliefs are well rooted in past medical and folk beliefs, but prevention is the first and best key to avoiding constipation. Cleansing enemas or laxatives are not the answer. Subsequently, you will find a list of common causes of constipation. It is important to discuss any bowel problems with the physician or nurse so that a proper evaluation can be completed. Guessing the cause of these problems should be avoided because some of them are quite serious.

- Low-fiber diet
- Dehydration (low fluid balance)
- Poor toileting habits
- Laxative abuse
- Immobility
- Loss of appetite (anorexia)
- Irritable bowel syndrome
- Depression
- Confusion
- Hemorrhoids
- Diabetes

- Low thyroid
- Cancer
- Drug therapy

The following are ways to avoid constipation naturally:

- Add fresh fruits and vegetables to the daily diet.
- Cut back on any highly processed foods, especially sweets, and avoid foods that are high in fat.
- Stay active.
- Drink 6 to 8 glasses of water daily. Fill a 2-quart pitcher each morning, and keep it in the refrigerator.
- Add unprocessed bran to items being baked and cereals.
- Provide privacy for toileting needs.
- Use a schedule for toileting.

DIARRHEA

Diarrhea needs to be evaluated by the physician and the underlying cause needs to be corrected. However, simple measures can also help. Improving the consistency of the stool can be helped along by the use of foods, such as rice, bananas, apples, yogurt, cheese, marshmallows, and some wheat products.

The following are common causes of fecal incontinence:

- Fecal impaction
- Laxative overuse abuse
- Neurological disorders, such as stroke
- Illnesses leading to diarrhea
- Rectal sphincter damage
- Nerve damage of diabetes (diabetic neuropathy)

The problem of fecal incontinence must always be evaluated by the physician. If the physician feels that this is a chronic condition (typically related to nervous system disorders, such as Alzheimer's disease), some helpful actions follow:

- Set up a toileting schedule.
- Physically assist the person to the toilet following a meal.
- Give praise for successes.
- Make sure the person is comfortable on the commode. You should assure privacy and physical warmth.
- Review the diet, and make sure there are not sources of GI irritation, such as overly spicy foods, lack of fiber, and so on.
- Remove any obvious sources of problems, such as laxatives.

Intestinal Gas

Intestinal gas is something that may also be troubling. It is believed that some foods tend to increase gas. You may want to limit these foods. They include foods, such as cabbage, wheat germ, onions, raisins, beans, and peas.

HYGIENE

The proper washing technique of the perianal area ("bottom") following toilet use is especially important for women. Washing and wiping oneself following toileting should be from the front to the back. Once a cloth or toilet paper has been used to wipe the anal or rectal area, it should not be passed back again over the front, vaginal area. The reason for this care is simple. Bacteria that normally live in bowel movement are not friendly when they contact the urinary tract. That is what happens if you wipe yourself from back to front. These bacteria can easily move up the urethra into the bladder and start infection.

A critical need for the person with urinary or fecal incontinence is to maintain clean, skin. After the bowel movement or incontinence (urinary or fecal), skin should be thoroughly washed with a nonirritating soap and dried. For urinary incontinence only, water may work fine. There are also commercially available products specifically for washing the perianal area. Use products that do not contain alcohol because this has a tendency to dry the skin.

Skin needs to be observed daily for any signs of breakdown. Beginning breakdown is easily recognized by redness and peeling away of layers of skin. Any rash should be reported to the physician or nurse. Various skin infections commonly occur as a result of continuous moisture in the perianal area.

CLOTHING

Clothing should be comfortable, attractive, and easy to manipulate. Styles that are especially popular are jogging-style suits with elastic waist and pull over shirts. The advantage of this clothing in addition to the ease and comfort of wearing and laundering, is that all age groups wear this type of clothing. Women also find dresses and skirts comfortable because of the ease for toileting. Though it may seem more convenient, bed clothing should be saved just for nighttime. Assisting the person to get up and get dressed helps preserve some of the normal aspects of day-to-day life that are helpful in maintaining function.

Women should avoid wearing nylon panties. Cotton is the best fabric for panties because it allows the skin to breathe. Toilet paper and sanitary napkins should be fragrance free.

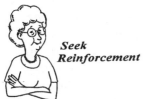

Seek Reinforcement

It is important to emphasize a few points. The information provided here is quite detailed and lengthy. The reason for this is simple. The bowel and bladder systems have been neglected for a long time, probably because of society's attitudes. Although we hear quite a bit about arthritis and heart disease, we do not hear much about incontinence. So it takes more "leg work" to catch people up on some of the basic information. If you are not interested in all the details, try to hit the highlights. The most important part is that you begin to look at bladder and bowel problems in a way that allows you to try new approaches. Not all bladder and bowel problems are "hopeless" or "inevitable." Many of them are very manageable.

Remember the team concept, "Together we can manage." Use all the resources you can find. Contact the national organizations and get on their mailing lists. Talk about incontinence with your health care team.

If bladder/bowel problems develop, try some of the simple measures first. Many people have fewer incontinence episodes by simply following dietary guidelines with adequate fluids, fiber, and exercise and a scheduled toileting program. It is very helpful to start with smaller steps. For example, if you have completed the bladder diary and find that the person has 10 episodes of incontinence each day, but is getting inadequate fluids, set your goal to correct the fluid problems first. Set up small steps toward that goal over a period of several weeks. Remember, the dependent older adult may not be able to adapt to quick changes. Also remember to reward successes when goals are reached.

10

Living and Dying with Dignity

Ann McCracken

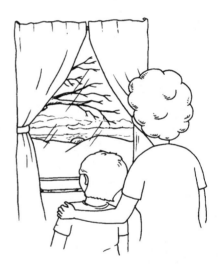

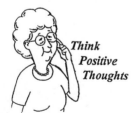

Think Positive Thoughts

Every loss that we experience brings with it the opportunity for personal growth and a chance to be a teacher to others by the way we respond to the loss. The author of this chapter shares some thoughts about her growth as she participated in her mother's dying experience.

The day before my mother died I sat on her hospital bed holding her hand. "You think I'm going to die, don't you?" she asked, looking straight at me. "Yes, Mom," I answered. "I think we are all going to die, but I think you are going to die before the rest of us." I continued on, reminding my mother of recent discussions we had of the dying process, . . . about it not being an unpleasant experience and that often there was a beautiful light and music. My mother interrupted, "My music will be country western." I nodded in total agreement.

I continued on, telling her that there is usually a person or deity to help the person pass over. I reminded her that I thought that the person for her would be my father, who had always been there for her in life until his untimely death at 56. "You have our messages for him, don't you?" I asked. She nodded as she drifted to some far off place where I could not follow. Her infrequent breathing reminded my brother and me of the finality of our watch. In the background, country music played on mom's favorite radio station as it had night and day for the past week. We waited, talking quietly in the twilight of an early summer evening.

It was nearly 2 hours later when she stirred, and our attention was drawn to the tiny figure in the bed. Slowly mom's eyes opened, searched the room to find us, and then she winked. "Fooled you!" she said, delighted that for this evening she had missed the connection to her distant journey. My mother, brother, and I joined in a communion of laughter that filled the room and overflowed into the world beyond.

CHALLENGE OF CHANGE

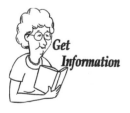
Get Information

Perhaps the one thing that we can count on in life is change. When we change, we gain something new, and we lose something familiar. The experience resembles the changing of clothes in one's closet for the season. To make room for the addition of a few up-to-date articles, you may need to take some seldom-worn clothes to the Goodwill store. This task is not an easy one because familiar memories are connected to those clothes. With life changes, too, we plunge ahead, often leaving behind some of the familiar. Our choice is to look longingly behind at that which was or to look ahead to the wonder of what is before us.

Aging brings with it an opportunity to perfect our response to change. At no time in life are there so many profound changes. Changes in vision, hearing, energy, lifestyles, support systems, and relationships offer opportunities to use coping skills acquired over a lifetime. We are also challenged to learn some new skills and incorporate new information into our lives. This chapter addresses perhaps the most difficult change—the process of dying and the death of a loved one. Although the content is primarily intended for the family caregiver and the dying family member, the information is also important for formal caregivers working closely with the family.

COPING WITH LOSS

Kubler-Ross, a well-known psychiatrist, observed that people who were dying worked through the loss of their life in a series of five stages: *denial, anger, bargaining, depression,* and *acceptance.* Caregivers of dying persons go through similar stages.

In *denial,* people deny they have a problem. They may look for doctors who will agree with them or they may decide not to follow treatments. In *anger,* they are angry at the world in general and doctors and other health care professionals in particular. It is important to remember that the root of the anger is the loss they are experiencing. In *bargaining,* they try to stave off the loss with promises, especially to God. "If only I recover I will—" is a bargaining approach.

Depression is a response to knowing that the loss is a reality. During this time, dying people should not be told to "look at the sunny side" or be given false hope. To do so would invalidate their feelings of loss. Just sitting together in silence is often effective. People need to mourn the impending death before they can move on to *acceptance* of death. People pass through these stages in different ways. The order may vary, and some people may repeat a stage.

ADVANCE DIRECTIVES

Discussing advance directives can be very difficult. Even when my mother had a terminal heart condition, I managed to avoid the subject.

One day I received a telephone call from her doctor in an emergency room over 500 miles away. He was calling to tell me that my mother was in a bout of congestive heart failure and was not responding to treatment. He wanted to know if they should do cardiopulmonary resuscitation whether my mother's heart stopped or if they should put her on a ventilator (a mechanical breathing device). I had no idea what my mother would have wanted me to do. Fortunately, in the 9 hours it took me to drive to the hospital, my mother had responded and was in cardiac intensive care. The next morning, with living will in hand, I told my mother that I always wanted to make the decisions that she would want me to make, but if I didn't know what she wanted, I would be unable to make them.

Quality of life has been defined in many ways. Having a purpose and making one's own decisions are often mentioned as important. Basically, it boils down to what makes a person feel that life is worth living. It differs from one person to another. Most people want to be in control of their health care decisions. Advance directives are used for this purpose. Advance directives are instructions to family and physicians and nurses about the health care preferences of people. The living will, medical power of attorney, and court-appointed guardianship are common ways in which caregivers make decisions for their loved ones who can no longer make decisions for themselves.

LIVING WILL

Living wills are directions to health care workers and family that are made in advance of actually needing them. Basically, a living will describes what types of treatment will be given to persons who have terminal conditions, with no chance of recovery. If the patient's wishes are not known, aggressive treatment, such as cardiopulmonary resuscitation (CPR, or mouth-to-mouth breathing and pressing down on the chest) is the standard procedure if the heart stops. This treatment occurs despite the fact that most older people do not survive despite CPR. Calling 911 means that everything possible will be done to resuscitate the patient.

Living will law varies from state to state. Calling the local office of ProSeniors, the local Area Agency on Aging, or the AARP can give you guidance in finding the appropriate forms. The living will covers treatments, such as CPR, tube feedings, and intravenous feedings (nutrition through the veins).

Once the living will is signed, it is important to give copies of the living will to the physician and to family members. A copy should be kept in an accessible place in the house in case it is needed in an emergency. If you are admitted to the hospital or a nursing home, the physician will write a "do not resuscitate order" on the chart, if it is requested in the living will. It would also be good to have a copy of your living will on the chart as well.

MEDICAL POWER OF ATTORNEY

Medical power of attorney is a document that authorizes whoever you name to make health care decisions for you in the event you are unable to speak for yourself. A medical power of attorney establishes a person to act on your behalf and gives that person the authority to make to all medical decisions for you. As with the living will, state laws differ. Current information on medical power of attorney in all states can be obtained from Concern for Dying/Society for the Right to Die, 250 West 57th Street, New York, NY 10107; telephone: (212) 246-6962 or 6973.

Some states have health care proxy laws. A health care proxy has the same authority to make health care decisions for a designated person as the medical power of attorney. The main difference is that a lawyer is not needed to complete the preprinted form. A local hospital or Area Agency on Aging can provide information about a state's health care proxy law and where to get the required form.

GUARDIANSHIP

A court may appoint a guardian for a person who is unable to make his or her own decisions and does not have a living will or a medical power of attorney. The guardian then makes decisions regarding the person and the person's estate the person's best interest or as the person would have made them. The guardian considers benefits, risks, and alternatives.

To become a guardian, a family caregiver would need to go through the court system to have the person declared legally incompetent and to be appointed as guardian. This process is much more involved than the living will and the medical power of attorney.

The guardian has to second guess what the person would have wanted if there are no explicit instructions about the person's choices.

Every adult should have a living will and medical power of attorney. In addition to having copies of these documents, it is also important to have together information on all legal, financial, and other important papers, such as wills, deeds, birth and marriage certificates, social security, mortgage, investment, checking, and savings accounts.

The following are key points for the caregiver to remember:

Problem. I want to carry out the health care wishes of the person I am caring for when he or she is not physically able to make decisions.

Goal. To have a written living will and medical power of attorney appropriate for the state in which the person for whom I am caring lives.

Actions. The following are specific actions to take:

- Discuss health care choices with the person(s) for whom you are caring, while they are still able to describe their preferences.
- Contact Concern for Dying/Society for the Right to Die, 250 West 57th Street, New York, NY 10107. Telephone (212) 246-6962 or 6973 and ask for the living will and medical power of attorney forms for the appropriate state. If they do not have the proper forms, call the local legal aid services or the Area Agency on Aging, or the AARP at (800)-434-3219 and ask for help in securing these forms.
- Help the person receiving your care as needed in completing the living will and the medical power of attorney forms.
- Make 5 to 10 copies of the living will and medical power of attorney, and give copies to family members and doctor. Have copies of these documents ready to take to the hospital or a nursing home if the person needs to be admitted.

Accomplishments. Congratulations! You are better prepared to make health care decisions.

DYING WITH DIGNITY

Like birth, death is one of the universal events for all human beings. Many persons are affected by the birth or death of one human being. Death with dignity is a fundamental right of all people.

Because dying persons have limited energy and strength, it is often the caregivers who are advocates for their rights. Decisions about the course of treatment for persons with terminal illnesses are not always clear-cut. One option is the *aggressive course*, which may only offer false hope of cure. If the patient is subjected to endless blood tests, biopsies, and other tests, the caregiver may need to decide whether the tests and treatments are really necessary. Three questions that caregivers have found helpful in making these decisions are the following:

1. What new information will the test provide?
2. How will the treatment change with this new information?
3. If treatment changes, will it change the outcome of the illness?

The basic question to ask about the use of aggressive treatment for a person with a terminal illness is, "Is the objective of treatment to prolong *life* or to prolong *dying*?" When death is imminent, one may want to switch the focus from noneffective "cure" to care and comfort. The dignity of dying persons can be maintained by giving them control and continued involvement in life.

My mother's physician was a wise and caring man. When it was apparent that my mother was going to die, her physician moved her from the cardiac intensive care unit to a private room where we could be with her at all times. Her physician also told her he would prescribe her usual medications as well as medication for anxiety and pain. He told her that she was in charge, and that she could decide what pills or treatments she wanted to take.

We continued to involve my mother in life. One week before her death, my daughter graduated from high school. Mom, who was her greatest fan, was very disappointed to miss this event. Five days before her death, however, she was able to see a videotape of the graduation with my daughter by her side. She was also able to give my daughter the quilt, sheets, and towels that would grace her room at college after her grandmother's death.

Each day we asked my mother what she would like to accomplish that day. Then we set about making that happen. One day it was to get a pepperoni pizza, most of which was eaten by the hospital staff. The day before she died, my mother wanted to pay her bills. Although the task took most of the day with many rest periods, she personally wrote and signed every check while we prepared the envelopes. The day of my mother's death, she wanted to see two friends who were invited and came to visit. She drifted in and out of the conversation during the short visit, but she seemed genuinely satisfied to have seen these good friends.

With a system of supportive family, many family caregivers are able to provide care until death. Others may choose to use other home caregivers or hospice resources. Hospice is a system of care that supports care and comfort for a person judged to have 6 months or less of life remaining. With the experience of many years of working with families, hospice staff can suggest ways to control pain, carry out daily activities, and live each day with the highest quality possible.

Hospices are listed in the yellow pages of the telephone book. It is good to find one that family or friends have found to be helpful and that has a long history of service in the local area. The National Hospice Organization can be reached at (800)-658-8898.

Dying persons have the right to be treated as human beings. They have the rights to make their own decisions and to receive truthful answers to their questions. Sometimes when a person has a terminal illness, people talk in the room as though they were not there. Research studies have shown that people hear, even when they appear to be in a coma.

One of the questions families seem to agonize over is whether or not to tell dying persons that they are dying. It is important to answer questions honestly. Knowing that one is dying certainly influences decisions and priorities. Perhaps even more important is the wall that divides people who are maintaining a deception. How lonely people must feel when they cannot discuss their death with those they love. In knowing the truth, dying persons can share their feelings about death and seek help from family; friends; and a minister, priest, or rabbi. A source of consolation to many people is their religious faith. Supporting them in their spiritual journey is important. Dying does not make troublesome relationships trouble free. It does, however, offer an opportunity for resolution and closure.

The following are key points for the caregiver to remember:

Problem. Making sure that the person I am caring for will get the best care possible.

Goals. The person I am caring for will

- Get care and treatments that maintain comfort and quality of life.
- Be involved in decisions and have health care wishes carried out.

Actions.
- Ask the doctor explain the tests, treatments, and the outcome in words that I understand.
- Tell the doctor to order only those tests that will change the treatment and the outcome.
- If the person is not comfortable, discuss this with the medical personnel. Call the National Hospice Organization at (800)-658-8898, and ask them for a local hospice that can be consulted for pain control.
- Ask medical personnel for things the person needs and wants if the person is in the hospital; be polite but firm.
- Ask the dying person what he or she would like to accomplish each day.
- Have available copies of the living will and the medical power of attorney; consult with the physician/nurses about what needs to be done and who to call at the time of death.

Congratulations—you have a plan! If you are not satisfied or need help, ask for Hospice Services. You can also call the local Area Agency on Aging or the AARP. If you find difficulty in legal issues like having the living will followed, check with your local legal aid services for seniors. If the person is in a nursing home, ask for the number of the ombudsman for the nursing home and call that person.

CAREGIVER AND GRIEVING

The ceremonies that surround the wake, funeral, memorial service, or scattering of ashes are society's way of supporting a grieving family. At one time, the family was very involved in all aspects of the funeral. Today much is left to the funeral director. Family involvement can be a way of beginning to work out the grieving process.

Feelings of sadness, anger, and emptiness are all a normal part of the grieving process. Insomnia, weight loss, and lack of energy are common physical symptoms that are experienced by grieving persons. Sharing your feelings of grief with others may be helpful. Support from family and friends is beneficial. Some people find it useful to join a support group of others who are working through the death of a loved one. Many people relate that their faith is the source of their strength.

Hospice grief counseling services are available to the caregiver for a year after the death of the person. Grieving takes time, however; if grief persists and remains intense for longer than 2 years, professional intervention is needed.

The AARP also has a free booklet titled *On Being Alone: Survival Handbook for Widows*. You can also call the Eldercare Locator at (800) 677-1116 for Bereavement Support Groups.

My mother's funeral involved input from sisters and brothers and grandchildren. I wrote and delivered the personalized eulogy that only a family member could. My daughter did a reading. Each of the grandchildren placed mementos under the silken cover that blanketed mother. In addition, they made sure that she had her coveted "bingo bag" just in case bingo was also a passion of the Almighty. Mom's dress and roses were red, her favorite color. When all was said and done, we each believed that Mom could not have had a better send-off and that we had a part in making that happen. In working together, we had begun our own journey to healing.

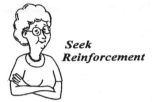

Seek Reinforcement

All of life is change. We spend a lifetime learning how to grow in the midst of change. The grieving process is a time of transition during which we learn to use the essence of what went before as the foundation for our new and different life. It is a time of intense personal pain that, when accepted, can lead to growth.

Chiam Potok in his book, *My Name is Asher Lev,* pointed out that what we have forever is never precious. Death reminds us that life is very precious. The death of a person we love is both the profound emptiness of loss and the celebration of a life that has profoundly changed our own.

Formal caregivers can help the family, particularly the family caregiver, with the grieving process. The family caregiver has lost a loved one but still has a life to be lived. Although it is good to stop and regroup by grieving the person who has died and reminiscing about the life shared, it is also important for the family caregiver to go forward with life.

The family caregiver needs to think about, "What will I do to have quality in my life after the death of my loved one?" Family caregivers and other caregivers need to give themselves permission to grieve and think about both the good times and the challenges shared with the person for whom they cared. The family caregiver needs to accept support from family and friends. Finally, the caregiver needs to decide the path he or she wants life to go, dream a new dream, and take responsibility for making the dream become real.

Appendix: Organizations and Resources

FOR GENERAL INFORMATION

Eldercare Locator
(800) 677-1116

Aging Network Services
4400 East West Highway
Suite 907
Bethesda, MD 20814
(301) 657-4329

American Association of Homes and Services for the Aging
1050 Seventeenth Street NW
Suite 770
Washington, DC 20036
(202) 783-2242

American Association of Retired Persons
601 E. Street NW
Washington, DC 20049
(800) 424-3410

American College of Sports Medicine
P.O. Box 1440
Indianapolis, IN 46206-1440
(317) 637-9200, ext. 117

Consumer Information Catalogue Services
P.O. Box 100
Pueblo, CO 81002
(719) 948-3334

Independent Living Aids
(800) 537-2118

National Association of Area Agencies on Aging
1112 16th Street NW, Suite 100
Washington, DC 20049
(800) 677-1116

National Council on the Aging
409 Third Street SW
Washington, DC 20024
(202) 479-1200

National Council of Senior Citizens
1331 F Street NW
Washington, DC 20004
(202) 347-8800

National Institute on Aging Information Center
P.O. Box 8057
Gaithersburg, MD 20898
(800) 222-2225

Sears Home Health Care
(800) 326-1750

U.S. Consumer Product Safety Commission
Washington, DC 20207
(800) 638-2772

FOR SPECIFIC PROBLEMS/QUESTIONS

ALCOHOL AND DRUG PROBLEMS

Alcoholics Anonymous
P.O. Box 459
Grand Central Station
New York, NY 10163
(212) 870-3400

ALZHEIMER'S DISEASE

Alzheimer's Association
919 N. Michigan Avenue
Suite 1000
Chicago, IL 60611
(800) 272-3900

Alzheimer's Disease Education
and Referral Center
P.O. Box 8250
Sliver Spring, MD 20907
(800) 438-4380

ARTHRITIS AND OSTEOPOROSIS

Arthritis Foundation
Information Line
P.O. Box 19000
Atlanta, GA 30326
(800) 283-7800

National Arthritis and Musculoskeletal and
   Skin Disease
Information Clearinghouse
1 AMS Circle
Bethesda, MD 20892
(301) 495-4484

National Arthritis Foundation
1909 Fort Myer Drive, Suite 507
Arlington, VA 22209
(703) 276-7555

National Osteoporosis Foundation
1150 17th Street NW Suite 500
Washington, DC 20036
(800) 223-9994 or (202) 223-2226

CANCER

American Cancer Society
1599 Clifton Road NE
Atlanta, GA 30329
(800) 227-2345
(404) 320-3333

Cancer Information Services
National Cancer Institute
Building 31, Room 10A24
Bethesda, MD 20892
(800) 422-6237

DEATH AND DYING

Concern for Dying/Society for the Right to Die
250 West 57th Street
New York, NY 10107
(212) 246-6962

Choice in Dying: Legal Forms
200 Varick St.
New York, NY 10014
(800) 989-9455

DIABETES

American Association of Diabetes Educators
444 N. Michigan Avenue, Suite 1240
Chicago, IL 60611
(800) 338-3633

American Diabetes Association
1660 Duke Street
Alexandria, VA 22314
(800) 232-3472

National Diabetes Information Clearinghouse
1 Information Way
Bethesda, MD 20892
(301) 654-3327

HEARING AND SPEECH

10801 Rockville Pike
Rockville, MD 20853
(301) 897-8682
(800) 638-8228

HEART DISEASE

American Heart Association
7272 Greenville Avenue
Dallas, TX 75231
(800) 242-1793

National Heart, Lung, and Blood Institute
Information Center
P.O. Box 30105
Bethesda, MD 20824-0105
(301) 251-1222

National Institute on Aging
Information Center
P.O. Box 8057
Gaithersburg, MD 20898-8057
(800) 222-2225

HOSPICE CARE

The National Hospice Organization
(800) 658-8898

INCONTINENCE

Alliance for Aging Research
2021 K Street NW, Suite 305
(202) 293-2856

Bladder Health Council
c/o American Foundation for Urologic Disease
300 West Pratt Street, Suite 401
Baltimore, MD 21201
(410) 727-2908

National Association for Continence
P.O. Box 8310
Spartanburg, SC 29305
(800) BLADDER
(800) 252-3337

Simon Foundation for Continence
Box 835
Wilmette, IL 60091
(800) 23-SIMON
(800) 237-4666

LEGAL AND FINANCIAL ISSUES

Legal Counsel for the Elderly
American Association of Retired Persons
(800) 424-3410

Medicare Rights Center
(212) 869-3850, ext. 19

Social Security Administration
(800) 772-1213

MENTAL HEALTH AND SUPPORT GROUPS

National Foundation for Depressive Illness
P.O. Box 2257
New York, NY 10116
(800) 248-4381

NUTRITION AND MEAL SERVICES

Food and Nutrition Information Center
National Agricultural Library
10301 Baltimore Boulevard, Room 304
Beltsville, MD 20705
(301) 344-3719

National Meals on Wheels Foundation
2675 44th Street SW, Suite 305
Grand Rapids, MI 49509
(800) 999-6262

Nutrition Hotline
American Dietetic Association
216 West Jackson Boulevard, Suite 800
Chicago, IL 60606
(800) 366-1655

PARKINSON'S DISEASE

American Parkinson's Disease Association
60 Bay Street Room 401
Staten Island, NY 10301
(800) 223-2732

STROKE

National Stroke Association
8480 E. Orchard Road, Suite 1000
Englewood, CO 80111
(800) 787-6537

VISION

American Council for the Blind
1010 Vermont Avenue NW
Suite 1100
Washington, DC 20005
(202) 393-3666
(800) 424-8666

American Council of the Blind
1155 15th Street NW, Suite 720
Washington, DC 20005
(800) 424-8866

American Foundation for the Blind
15 West 16th Street
New York, NY 10011
(212) 620-2039

INTERNET RESOURCES FOR CAREGIVERS

ADMINISTRATION ON AGING: INFORMATION FOR OLDER PERSONS
AND THEIR FAMILIES

URL: http://www.aoa.dhhs.gov/elderpage.html

ELDERCARE LOCATOR

URL: http://www.state.me.us/beas/locator.htm

FAMILY CAREGIVER ALLIANCE

URL: http://www.caregiver.org

FREE STUFF—THE SENIORS' YELLOW PAGES—DESCRIPTIONS OF ORGANIZATIONS

URL: http://www.thirdage.com/freestuff/yellow/ch19_89.html

MEDICARE ASSISTANCE PLAN

URL: http://www.medicarerights.org

SENIOR NET

URL: http://www.seniornet.org

SENIOR LINK

URL: http://www.seniorlink.com

SENIOR LAW

URL: http://www.seniorlaw.com

TRANSPORTATION

URL: http://www.aarporg/programs/transportation/transwhom. html

Index

S *Springer Publishing Company*

What Every Home Health Nurse Needs to Know, Volume 2
A Book of Readings

Majorie McHann, RN, BS

A perfect complement to book one, this compilation of thirty new readings addresses the changing role of the home health nurse with an emphasis on such relevant concerns as outcomes management, legal issues, and strategies for success. Maintaining a hands-on approach, readings were selected for their immediate usefulness addressing such basic issues as how to be "street smart"; how to be a"guest" in the patient's home; master skilled documentation and Medicare intricacies.

1998   191pp   0-8261-9131-2   softcover

What Every Home Health Nurse Needs to Know, Volume 1
A Book of Readings

Majorie McHann, RN, BS

An anthology of practical, down-to-earth readings on home care nursing from a range of journals, books, and video transcripts. Readings were selected for their immediate usefulness to clinicians on topics such as medicare coverage, skilled documentation, clinical management, patient education, quality assurance, and legal issues. A valuable resource for students, practicing nurses, and home care administrators.

1998   210pp   0-8261-9130-4   softcover
Volume 1 & 2 Set   0-8261-9132-0

536 Broadway, New York, NY 10012-3955 • (212) 431-4370 • Fax (212) 941-7842

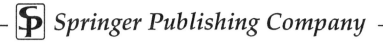

Springer Publishing Company

Making the Transition to Home Health Nursing
A Practical Guide
Denise Lovejoy, RN, MS

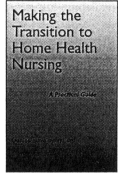

A practical orientation to the world of home care nursing, this volume is for new nurse graduates and hospital nurses who wish to change to home care. Coming from the tightly structured world of the hospital, nurses may find the responsibilities, freedom, initiative, and ever-changing patient environment of home care both exhilarating and intimidating.

This book, written by an experienced home health nurse, provides a wealth of practical tips and information, including a description of how a home health agency operates, how to develop time and case management skills, how to arrange for peer support, and the nuts and bolts of a typical home health care visit. Includes a valuable and extensive appendix on Medicare eligibility rules and regulations.

Contents:

Understanding Home Care
- Home Care vs. Hospital Nursing —A Comparison
- Home Care Structure
- Adapting to the Home Care Setting

Making the Home Visit: From Preparation to Completion
- Before the Visit
- During the Visit
- After the Visit

Important Issues in Caseload Management
- Physical Characteristics of Home Care Environment
- People's Homes
- On The Road
- Appendices

1997   188pp   0-8261-9740-X   hardcover

536 Broadway, New York, NY 10012-3955 • (212) 431-4370 • Fax (212) 941-7842

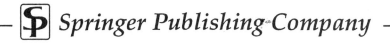

Springer Publishing Company

Guardianship of the Elderly
Psychiatric and Judicial Aspects

George H. Zimny, PhD
George T. Grossberg, MD
Foreword **Jessie A. Goldner**

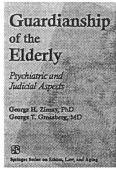

This book provides a basic explanation of guardianship of elderly persons and the process by which it takes place. Through contributions by geriatric psychiatrists, psychologists, attorneys, and judges, this volume provides a basic understanding of what can occur before, during, and after guardianship.This concise volume reviews all aspects of the guardianship process and provides new insights to insure that the future development of guardianship is in a direction that makes it as humane and effective as possible. This book is a valuable guide to students and members of disciplines and organizations involved with the care of elderly persons including: social work, gerontology, law, medicine, psychology, nursing, and finance.

Contents:

1998   155pp   0-8261-1176-9   softcover

536 Broadway, New York, NY 10012-3955 • (212) 431-4370 • Fax (212) 941-7842